Progress in Behavioral Health Interventions for Children and Adolescents

Editors

XIAOMING LI
SAYWARD HARRISON

PEDIATRIC CLINICS
OF NORTH AMERICA

www.pediatric.theclinics.com

Consulting Editor
BONITA F. STANTON

August 2022 • Volume 69 • Number 4

ELSEVIER

1600 John F. Kennedy Boulevard • Suite 1800 • Philadelphia, Pennsylvania, 19103-2899

http://www.theclinics.com

THE PEDIATRIC CLINICS OF NORTH AMERICA Volume 69, Number 4
August 2022 ISSN 0031-3955, ISBN-13: 978-0-323-98717-2

Editor: Kerry Holland
Developmental Editor: Axell Ivan Jade M. Purificacion

The Pediatric Clinics of North America (ISSN 0031-3955) is published bimonthly by Elsevier Inc., 360 Park Avenue South, New York, NY 10010-1710. Months of issue are February, April, June, August, October, and December. Periodicals postage paid at New York, NY and additional mailing offices. Subscription prices are $263.00 per year (US individuals), $1028.00 per year (US institutions), $331.00 per year (Canadian individuals), $1074.00 per year (Canadian institutions), $395.00 per year (international individuals), $1074.00 per year (international institutions), $100.00 per year (US students and residents), $100.00 per year (Canadian students and residents), and $165.00 per year (international residents and students). To receive students/resident rare, orders must be accompanied by name of affiliated institution, date of term, and the signature of program/residency coordinator on institution letterhead. Orders will be billed at individual rate until proof of status is received. Foreign air speed delivery is included in all Clinics subscription prices. All prices are subject to change without notice. **POSTMASTER: Send address changes to The Pediatric Clinics of North America,** Elsevier Health Sciences Division, Subscription Customer Service, 3251 Riverport Lane, Maryland Heights, MO 63043. **Customer Service: 1-800-654-2452 (US and Canada). From outside of the US and Canada: 1-314-447-8871. Fax: 1-314-447-8029. For print support, E-mail: JournalsCustomerService-usa@elsevier. com. For online support, E-mail: JournalsOnlineSupport-usa@elsevier.com.**

Reprints. For copies of 100 or more, of articles in this publication, please contact the Commercial Reprints Department, Elsevier Inc., 360 Park Avenue South, New York, NY 10010-1710. Tel.: 212-633-3874; Fax: 212-633-3820; E-mail: reprints@elsevier.com.

The Pediatric Clinics of North America is also published in Spanish by McGraw-Hill Inter-americana Editores S.A., Mexico City, Mexico; in Portuguese by Riechmann and Affonso Editores, Rua Comandante Coelho 1085, CEP 21250, Rio de Janeiro, Brazil; and in Greek by Althayia SA, Athens, Greece.

The Pediatric Clinics of North America is covered in MEDLINE/PubMed (Index Medicus), Excerpta Medica, Current Contents, Current Contents/Clinical Medicine, Science Citation Index, ASCA, ISI/BIOMED, and BIOSIS.

PROGRAM OBJECTIVE

The goal of the *Pediatric Clinics of North America* is to keep practicing physicians and residents up to date with current clinical practice in pediatrics by providing timely articles reviewing the state-of-the-art in patient care.

TARGET AUDIENCE

All practicing pediatricians, physicians, and healthcare professionals who provide patient care to pediatric patients.

LEARNING OBJECTIVES

Upon completion of this activity, participants will be able to:

1. Review the risk factors that contribute to the health and behavior of children and the impact on families and caregivers.
2. Discuss the strategies, interventions, and theoretical frameworks that might be utilized to encourage children to improve their behavior and achieve positive outcomes for themselves, their families, and caregivers.
3. Recognize the importance of a multidisciplinary team and a collaborative care approach in providing effective care, providing support, and promoting positive outcomes for children, their families, and caregivers experiencing a variety of behavioral health issues.

ACCREDITATIONS

Physician Credit

The Elsevier Office of Continuing Medical Education (EOCME) is accredited by the Accreditation Council for Continuing Medical Education (ACCME) to provide continuing medical education for physicians.

The EOCME designates this journal-based activity for a maximum of 12 *AMA PRA Category 1 Credit*(s)™. Physicians should claim only the credit commensurate with the extent of their participation in the activity.

All other healthcare professionals requesting continuing education credit for this journal-based activity will be issued a certificate of participation.

ABP Maintenance of Certification Credit

Successful completion of this CME activity, which includes participation in the activity and individual assessment of and feedback to the learner, enables the learner to earn up to 12 MOC points in the American Board of Pediatrics' (ABP) Maintenance of Certification (MOC) program. It is the CME activity provider's responsibility to submit learner completion information to ACCME for the purpose of granting ABP MOC credit.

DISCLOSURE OF CONFLICTS OF INTEREST

The EOCME assesses conflict of interest with its instructors, faculty, planners, and other individuals who are in a position to control the content of CME activities. All relevant conflicts of interest that are identified are thoroughly vetted by EOCME for fair balance, scientific objectivity, and patient care recommendations. EOCME is committed to providing its learners with CME activities that promote improvements or quality in healthcare and not a specific proprietary business or a commercial interest.

The planning committee, staff, authors, and editors listed below have identified no financial relationships or relationships to products or devices they or their spouse/life partner have with commercial interest related to the content of this CME activity:

Elizabeth L. Adams, PhD; Bridget Armstrong, PhD; Michael Beets, PhD; Eric G. Benotsch, PhD; Jessica Bradshaw, PhD; Henna Budhwani, PhD, MPH; Darien Collins, BA; Brian P. Daly, PhD; Brian P. Daly, PhD; Taylor Davis, Ed.S; Kristen Figas, Ed.S; Paul Flaspohler, PhD; Nada M. Goodrum, PhD; Sara K. Shaw Green, MSW; Sayward Harrison, PhD; Caroline Hensing; Robert Hock, PhD; Yanping Jiang, PhD; Paul C. Jones, PhD; Jenna Kiely, BA; Amelia S. Knopf, PhD, MPH, RN, FAAN; Xiaoming Li, PhD; Shannon Litke, BA; Karen MacDonell, PhD; Kathryn Mancini, PhD; Kyle Liam Mason, MS; Rajkumar Mayakrishnan, BSc, MBA; Sylvie Naar, PhD; Ronald J. Prinz, PhD; Erin Scherder, Ed.S; Layne Scopano; Shelby A. Smout, MS; Kelly Stern, MA; Robert Stevens, PhD; Allison M. Sweeney, PhD; Cheuk Chi Tam, PhD; John Terry, PhD; Doreen Thomas-Payne, MSN, BSN, RN, PMHNP-BC; Catherine S.J. Wall, BS; Katelyn Wargel, MA, MPA; R. Glenn Weaver, PhD; Mark D. Weist, PhD; Dawn K. Wilson, PhD; Katie Wolfe, PhD; Nicole Zarrett, PhD

The planning committee, staff, authors and editors listed below have identified financial relationships or relationships to products or devices they or their spouse/life partner have with commercial interest related to the content of this CME activity:

Simone J. Skeen, MA: *Advisor*: Waverider

UNAPPROVED/OFF-LABEL USE DISCLOSURE

The EOCME requires CME faculty to disclose to the participants:

1. When products or procedures being discussed are off-label, unlabelled, experimental, and/or investigational (not US Food and Drug Administration [FDA] approved); and
2. Any limitations on the information presented, such as data that are preliminary or that represent ongoing research, interim analyses, and/or unsupported opinions. Faculty may discuss information about pharmaceutical agents that is outside of FDA-approved labelling. This information is intended solely for CME and is not intended to promote off-label use of these medications. If you have any questions, contact the medical affairs department of the manufacturer for the most recent prescribing information.

TO ENROLL

To enroll in the *Pediatric Clinics of North America* Continuing Medical Education program, call customer service at 1-800-654-2452 or sign up online at http://www.theclinics.com/home/cme. The CME program is available to subscribers for an additional annual fee of USD 324.00.

METHOD OF PARTICIPATION

In order to claim credit, participants must complete the following:

1. Complete enrolment as indicated above.
2. Read the activity.
3. Complete the CME Test and Evaluation. Participants must achieve a score of 70% on the test. All CME Tests and Evaluations must be completed online.

In order to claim MOC points, participants must complete the following:

1. Complete steps listed above for claiming CME credit
2. Provide your specialty board ID#, birth date (MM/DD), and attestation.
3. Online MOC submission is only available for the American Board of pediatrics' (ABP) Maintenance of Certification (MOC) program

CME INQUIRIES/SPECIAL NEEDS

For all CME inquiries or special needs, please contact elsevierCME@elsevier.com

Contributors

CONSULTING EDITOR

BONITA F. STANTON, MD
Professor of Pediatrics and Founding Dean, Robert C. and Laura C. Garrett Endowed Chair, Hackensack Meridian School of Medicine, President, Academic Enterprise, Hackensack Meridian Health, Nutley, New Jersey

EDITORS

XIAOMING LI, PhD
Professor and SmartState Endowed Chair for Clinical Translational Research, Department of Health Promotion, Education, and Behavior, South Carolina SmartState Center for Healthcare Quality, Arnold School of Public Health, University of South Carolina, Columbia, South Carolina

SAYWARD E. HARRISON, PhD
Assistant Professor, Department of Psychology, South Carolina SmartState Center for Healthcare Quality, Arnold School of Public Health, University of South Carolina, Columbia, South Carolina

AUTHORS

ELIZABETH L. ADAMS, PhD
Arnold School of Public Health, University of South Carolina, Columbia, South Carolina

BRIDGET ARMSTRONG, PhD
Arnold School of Public Health, University of South Carolina, Columbia, South Carolina

MICHAEL BEETS, PhD
Arnold School of Public Health, University of South Carolina, Columbia, South Carolina

ERIC G. BENOTSCH, PhD
Department of Psychology, Virginia Commonwealth University, Richmond, Virginia

JESSICA BRADSHAW, PhD
Assistant Professor, Carolina Autism and Neurodevelopment Research Center, University of South Carolina, Columbia, South Carolina

HENNA BUDHWANI, PhD, MPH
Department of Health Policy and Organization, University of Alabama at Birmingham (UAB), School of Public Health (SOPH), Birmingham, Alabama; Florida State University College of Medicine (FSU), Center for Translational Behavioral Science (CTBScience), Tallahassee, Florida

DARIEN COLLINS, BA
Department of Psychology, University of South Carolina, Barnwell College, Columbia, South Carolina

BRIAN P. DALY, PhD
Associate Professor and Department Head, Department of Psychological and Brain Sciences, Drexel University, Philadelphia, Pennsylvania

TAYLOR DAVIS, EdS
Department of Psychology, University of South Carolina, Barnwell College, Columbia, South Carolina

KRISTEN FIGAS, EdS
Department of Psychology, University of South Carolina, Barnwell College, Columbia, South Carolina

PAUL FLASPOHLER, PhD
Professor and Director of Research and Evaluation, Department of Psychology, Miami University, Oxford, Ohio

NADA M. GOODRUM, PhD
Assistant Professor, Department of Psychology, Research Center for Child Well-Being, University of South Carolina, Columbia, South Carolina

SAYWARD E. HARRISON, PhD
Assistant Professor, Department of Psychology, South Carolina SmartState Center for Healthcare Quality, Arnold School of Public Health, University of South Carolina, Columbia, South Carolina

CAROLINE HENSING
Arnold School of Public Health, University of South Carolina, Columbia, South Carolina

ROBERT HOCK, PhD
Associate Professor, Carolina Autism and Neurodevelopment Research Center, University of South Carolina, Columbia, South Carolina

YANPING JIANG, PhD
Institute for Health, Health Care Policy, and Aging Research, Department of Family Medicine and Community Health, Rutgers, The State University of New Jersey, New Brunswick, New Jersey

PAUL C. JONES, PhD
Assistant Professor, Psychological Studies in Education, Temple University, Philadelphia, Pennsylvania

JENNA KIELY, BA
Clinical Research Coordinator, PolicyLab and the Center for Pediatric Clinical Effectiveness, Children's Hospital of Philadelphia (CHOP), Philadelphia, Pennsylvania

KAREN KOLMODIN MACDONELL, PhD
Wayne State University School of Medicine, Family Medicine and Public Health Sciences, Detroit, Michigan

AMELIA S. KNOPF, PhD, MPH, RN
Community and Health Systems, Indiana University School of Nursing, Indianapolis, Indiana

XIAOMING LI, PhD
Professor and SmartState Endowed Chair for Clinical Translational Research, Department of Health Promotion, Education, and Behavior, South Carolina SmartState Center for Healthcare Quality, Arnold School of Public Health, University of South Carolina, Columbia, South Carolina

SHANNON LITKE, BA
Clinical Psychology Graduate Student, Department of Psychological and Brain Sciences, Drexel University, Philadelphia, Pennsylvania

KATHRYN MANCINI, PhD
Pediatric Psychologist, MetroHealth Medical Center, Assistant Professor, Case Western Reserve University School of Medicine, Cleveland Ohio

KYLE LIAM MASON, MS
Department of Psychology, Virginia Commonwealth University, Richmond, Virginia

SYLVIE NAAR, PhD
Florida State University College of Medicine (FSU), Center for Translational Behavioral Science (CTBScience), Tallahassee, Florida

RONALD J. PRINZ, PhD
Carolina Distinguished Professor, Department of Psychology, Research Center for Child Well-Being, University of South Carolina, Columbia, South Carolina

ERIN SCHERDER, EdS
Department of Psychology, University of South Carolina, Barnwell College, Columbia, South Carolina

LAYNE SCOPANO
University of South Carolina, Columbia, South Carolina

SARA K. SHAW GREEN, MSW
Center for Translational Behavioral Science, Florida State University, Tallahassee, Florida

SIMONE J. SKEEN, MA
Department of Social, Behavioral, and Population Sciences, School of Public Health and Tropical Medicine, Tulane University, New Orleans, Louisiana

SHELBY A. SMOUT, MS
Department of Psychology, Virginia Commonwealth University, Richmond, Virginia

KELLY STERN, MA
West Hawaii Complex Area, Hawaii School District, Kealakehe High School – SBBH Office, Kalua-Kona, Hawaii

ROBERT STEVENS, PhD
Department of Psychology, University of South Carolina, Barnwell College, Columbia, South Carolina

ALLISON M. SWEENEY, PhD
Assistant Professor, College of Nursing, University of South Carolina, Columbia, South Carolina

CHEUK CHI TAM, PhD
South Carolina SmartState Center for Healthcare Quality, Department of Health Promotion, Education, and Behavior, Arnold School of Public Health, University of South Carolina, Columbia, South Carolina

JOHN TERRY, PhD
Department of Psychology, University of South Carolina, Barnwell College, Columbia, South Carolina

CATHERINE S.J. WALL, BS
Department of Psychology, Virginia Commonwealth University, Richmond, Virginia

KATELYN WARGEL, MA, MPA
Clinical Psychology Graduate Student, Department of Psychology, Miami University, Oxford, Ohio

R. GLENN WEAVER, PhD
Arnold School of Public Health, University of South Carolina, Columbia, South Carolina

MARK D. WEIST, PhD
Department of Psychology, University of South Carolina, Barnwell College, Columbia, South Carolina

DAWN K. WILSON, PhD
Professor, Department of Psychology, Barnwell College, University of South Carolina, Columbia, South Carolina

KATIE WOLFE, PhD
Associate Professor, Carolina Autism and Neurodevelopment Research Center, University of South Carolina, Columbia, South Carolina

NICOLE ZARRETT, PhD
Professor, Department of Psychology, Barnwell College, University of South Carolina, Columbia, South Carolina

Contents

> Most children experience potentially traumatic events, and some develop significant emotional and behavioral difficulties in response. Although the field has mainly focused on treatment, a prevention framework provides an alternate approach to reducing the public health burden of trauma. Because parents and families can affect children's trauma exposure and reactions, family-based preventive interventions represent a unique opportunity to address child traumatic stress. This article discusses family-based programs that address child traumatic stress across 3 categories: preventing children's exposure to traumatic events, preventing traumatic stress reactions following exposure, and preventing negative long-term sequelae of trauma.

> The rising prevalence of autism spectrum disorder (ASD) calls for clear referral and treatment guidelines for children with ASD and their caregivers. Caregiver involvement in intervention is a standard practice of care and research suggests that teaching intervention strategies to caregivers can improve child outcomes and increase caregiver efficacy. Caregiver-mediated interventions that are naturalistic, developmental, and behavioral are effective in improving social and communication skills for children with ASD. Caregiver training models that use behavioral strategies are effective in reducing challenging behaviors. Finally, reducing caregiver barriers to treatment implementation, including stress and strain, are becoming critical components for improving the well-being and care of children with ASD and their families.

> We provide a transactional model of health for understanding the early risk of obesity in youth. This model argues that positive health is construed through the choices and actions that youth take within the range of resources and constraints of their biological and contextual situations across time. Social, cognitive, affective, and behavioral regulatory/motivational processes within the child mediate the relation between life experiences and health outcomes and obesity pathways are influenced by cumulative risk or protective processes for health promotion/compromising behaviors influencing health. We provide evidence-based examples of multilevel approaches to obesity prevention and treatment and highlight recommendations for future health behavior interventions.

Children's movement behaviors (ie, sedentary behaviors, physical activity, and sleep) are related to obesity risk and may vary throughout the year. The purpose of this systematic review is to summarize existing literature on the seasonal variation in physical activity and sleep in children. This study found that children's behaviors fluctuate seasonally and thus, interventions must target behaviors during the times when children's behaviors are the least healthy, specifically during the summer (when children are not in school) and winter. Finally, the paucity of data on seasonal variation in sleep indicates a need for further research in this area.

Across Western countries, approximately 15% to 20% of school-aged children and adolescents have a health-related disorder, with incidence rates of childhood chronic health conditions (CHCs) increasing. This contribution comprehensively reviews disease-level, school-level, and systems-level issues related to effectively supporting children with CHCs succeed from both psychosocial and educational perspectives. This article also delineates training needs as they pertain to graduate preparation and/or professional development to equip school personnel to appropriately address students' needs. The article concludes with recommendations for evidence-based prevention and intervention strategies and potential avenues for interdisciplinary collaboration and models of coordinated care for these medically compromised youth.

Integrating behavioral health care into pediatric primary care (PPC) settings can increase access to behavioral health promotion services and treatment. Efficient models for integrated PPC are emerging. Recent reviews call for integrated PPC research to better identify efficient teaming and processes, particularly in areas of building integrated PPC team member capacity and adopting practices that promote "upstream" behavioral wellness specific to community needs. Research in integrating behavioral health in schools has identified key practices relevant to these gaps in integrated primary care (IPC) research. This article discusses possibilities to apply findings from integrated school behavioral health research to IPC settings.

There is a national movement to advance school behavioral health, involving the mental health system partnering with schools' multitiered systems of support. This article underscores the critical need for school behavioral health and presents strategies to advance effective programming at district, state, and regional levels. Themes include diverse stakeholder involvement, teaming, data-based decision-making, implementation of evidence-based practices, screening, coaching and implementation support, progress monitoring and outcome evaluation, and using findings to scale-up effective programming. Implications for research, practice, and policy are reviewed along with ideas for the future development of this field.

Despite the continuing integration of digital outreach tools into adolescent preventive services, adaptive guidance for their ethical use remains limited. In this configurative review, we synthesize the ad hoc, applied digital bioethics developed in adolescent human immunodeficiency virus prevention science. By focusing on generalizable technological affordances, while balancing privacy and autonomy, we offer strategies for identifying potential technologically mediated harms that can transcend specific platforms, tools, or the knowledge levels of individual clinicians. Clinical vignettes illustrate the application of these strategies.

HIV is now a chronic condition that can be managed. Adolescents and emerging adults represent a large proportion of new diagnoses, but struggle with many aspects of HIV-related self-management. Self-management of HIV is critical to maintaining health and involves retention in HIV care, medication adherence to achieve viral suppression, managing substance use, and sexual and general health-related behaviors. This article describes theoretic frameworks for HIV self-management as adapted for youth and reviews self-management interventions developed to improve health outcomes in youth living with HIV identified from a recent systematic review.

Motivational Interviewing (MI) is a highly specified behavior change communication approach to improve patient–provider relationships, provider communication, and patient health outcomes. Because MI is built on a foundation of patient autonomy support, a feature known to positively influence behavior change during adolescence and emerging adulthood, MI is an evidence-based framework that can inform interventions targeting improvements in health outcomes among youth. MI can be difficult to implement with adequate fidelity, because learning MI requires time and commitment from busy providers with competing priorities. This review addresses best practices for implementing MI within adolescent serving medical settings (eg, pediatrics, family practices, rural health clinics, community health organizations, and so forth), including an orientation to MI, examples of efficacious interventions that were developed leveraging MI, and consideration for the design of training programs that include ongoing support to maximize the likelihood of sustainment.

The resilience framework offers a powerful tool to study how individuals respond to adversity. Intervention efforts building on 40 years of resilience research show promise in promoting mental and behavioral health of children in the context of adversity. This paper provides an overview of resilience and resilience-based interventions on mental and behavioral health in children. The importance of understanding resilience through the lens of the socioecological systems theory is highlighted, and the potential benefit of multilevel interventions in promoting mental and behavioral health is discussed.

The nonmedical use of prescription drugs (NMUPD) is a public health crisis. In 2020, more Americans died of drug overdose than in any prior year, and the nonmedical use of opioids and other prescription drugs contributed significantly to that total. Young adults and adolescents report the highest rates of NMUPD, relative to other age groups. This article provides a narrative review of interventions for young adults and adolescents to prevent NMUPD, including interventions directed at the individual, family or other small group, and community. The interventions reviewed included those that were delivered in person and via technology.

PEDIATRIC CLINICS OF NORTH AMERICA

SERIES OF RELATED INTEREST

Critical Care Clinics of North America
www.criticalcare.theclinics.com

THE CLINICS ARE AVAILABLE ONLINE!
Access your subscription at:
www.theclinics.com

Preface

Progress in Behavioral Health Interventions for Children and Adolescents

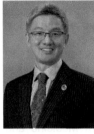 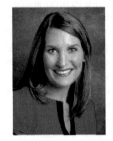

Xiaoming Li, PhD   Sayward Harrison, PhD
Editors

Prior to the onset of the COVID-19 pandemic, one in five children and adolescents in the United States experienced a mental, emotional, developmental, or behavioral health disorder each year,[1] with far too many unable to access evidence-based care. The pandemic has exacerbated these challenges in the United States and worldwide and has exposed stark disparities in access to and quality of behavioral health services for children and families. The urgency of the mental and behavioral health crisis among youth was highlighted in an advisory issued by the US Surgeon General in 2021 calling for a swift and coordinated response to support the mental and behavioral health needs of youth and families.[2]

Yet despite the extensive challenges created by the global pandemic, today there is a stronger body of evidence and more resources than ever before to meet these behavioral health needs. In addition, technological innovation and rapid proliferation of mobile health tools have expanded our ability to scale up behavioral health care in order to deliver timely and tailored services to those experiencing mental and behavioral health disorders. Similarly, the field of prevention science has proliferated in recent years—offering the opportunity to prevent many mental and behavioral health challenges before they ever develop. Despite these advances, pediatric providers often feel ill-equipped and underresourced to integrate the prevention and treatment of mental and behavioral health disorders into their practice—whether due to lack of knowledge, limited comfort, time constraints, competing demands, or other systems-level barriers.

This focused issue of *Pediatric Clinics of North America* has been curated to address this gap by synthesizing recent advances in pediatric behavioral health care across a variety of conditions frequently encountered in pediatric practice. Because pediatric

Pediatr Clin N Am 69 (2022) xv–xvi
https://doi.org/10.1016/j.pcl.2022.06.001
0031-3955/22/© 2022 Published by Elsevier Inc.

pediatric.theclinics.com

providers are often the first stop for concerned caregivers, staying abreast of developments in the prevention, diagnosis, and treatment of common mental and behavioral health disorders is critical.

In this issue, we present 12 articles that provide insight for addressing a range of behavioral health concerns in the general pediatric population as well as for specific patient groups. While the behavioral foci of included articles are wide ranging (ie, childhood obesity, self-management for youth with chronic health conditions, nonmedical use of prescription drugs among adolescents), all articles highlight the wealth of knowledge that exists to inform practical approaches to promote positive behavioral health and mental health among youth. We have taken care to emphasize the advantages of integrating behavioral health services into pediatric primary care settings. We also highlight the unique benefits of school-based behavioral and mental health care and the critical importance of engaging families across the prevention and treatment continuums.

While there is much work to be done to overcome the negative impacts of COVID-19 on the well-being of children and adolescents, this issue spurs hope that advances in our scientific understanding of effective behavioral health care will translate to greater health equity, particularly for youth from vulnerable and marginalized populations. On that note, we dedicate this issue to the late Bonita F. Stanton, MD (1951-2022), who served as founding dean of the Hackensack Meridian School of Medicine and Consulting Editor of *Pediatric Clinics of North America* for many years. Dr Stanton's remarkable career as a pediatrician, scientist, and visionary in medical education has left an indelible mark not only on the fields of medicine and public health but also on the countless lives that she touched along the way.

Xiaoming Li, PhD
Department of Health Promotion, Education, and Behavior
University of South Carolina
915 Greene Street
Discovery 1 Building, Suite #409
Columbia, SC 29208, USA

Sayward Harrison, PhD
Department of Psychology
University of South Carolina
1512 Pendleton Street
Barnwell College, Suite #220
Columbia, SC 29208, USA

E-mail addresses:
xiaoming@mailbox.sc.edu (X. Li)
harri764@mailbox.sc.edu (S. Harrison)

REFERENCES

1. Bitsko RH, Claussen AH, Lichstein J, et al. Mental health surveillance among children—United States, 2013–2019. MMWR 2022;71(2):1–42.
2. Office of the Surgeon General. US Surgeon General issues advisory on youth mental health crisis further exposed by COVID-19 pandemic. 2021. Available at: https://www.hhs.gov/about/news/2021/12/07/us-surgeon-general-issues-advisory-on-youth-mental-health-crisis-further-exposed-by-covid-19-pandemic.html. Accessed May 1, 2022.

Family-Based Prevention of Child Traumatic Stress

Nada M. Goodrum, PhD[a,b,*], Ronald J. Prinz, PhD[a,b]

KEYWORDS

- Prevention • Children • Adolescents • Trauma • Families • PTSD • Parenting
- Family-based intervention

KEY POINTS

- Most children are exposed to potentially traumatic events and some develop traumatic stress reactions including emotional and behavioral difficulties.
- Positive parenting and family support are key protective factors for children who have experienced or might experience potentially traumatic events.
- Family-based preventive interventions can address child traumatic stress by preventing children's exposure to traumatic events, traumatic stress reactions following exposure, and long-term negative sequelae of trauma.

CHILDHOOD TRAUMATIC STRESS

Exposure to potentially traumatic events (PTEs), unfortunately, is common in childhood, with nearly two-thirds of children experiencing at least one PTE before age 18 years.[1] Childhood PTEs can include child maltreatment (physical abuse, neglect, sexual abuse, emotional abuse), exposure to violence at home or in the community, serious accidents or injuries (eg, motor vehicle crashes), life-threatening illnesses or medical conditions, natural disasters, and sudden or violent death of a loved one. Although most children are resilient to these events or experience natural recovery from distress, about 1 in 6 PTE-exposed children develop clinically significant posttraumatic stress disorder (PTSD), with girls, children of color, and those exposed to interpersonal trauma at highest risk.[2–4] Children of color, especially Black/African American and Hispanic/Latino children, are more likely than their White peers to experience PTEs and to develop trauma-related mental health concerns, yet they are less likely to receive trauma-focused treatment.[3] These disparities may be partially due to pervasive and structural factors such as racial discrimination, unjustified mass

[a] Department of Psychology, University of South Carolina, 1512 Pendleton Street, Barnwell College, Suite #220, Columbia, SC 29208, USA; [b] Research Center for Child Well-Being, University of South Carolina, 1400 Pickens Street, Suite 400, Columbia, SC 29201, USA
* Corresponding author. Department of Psychology, University of South Carolina, 1512 Pendleton Street, Barnwell College, Suite #220, Columbia, SC 29208.
E-mail address: ngoodrum@mailbox.sc.edu

Pediatr Clin N Am 69 (2022) 633–644
https://doi.org/10.1016/j.pcl.2022.04.011
0031-3955/22/© 2022 Elsevier Inc. All rights reserved.

pediatric.theclinics.com

incarceration, and other forms of systemic racism that lead to unfavorable social conditions (eg, poverty), leaving children at higher risk of unaddressed traumatic stress.[5,6]

PTSD symptoms include intrusions such as unwanted memories, nightmares, or flashbacks; avoidance of trauma-related stimuli; negative thoughts or feelings such as self-blame and decreased interest in activities; and hyperarousal or reactivity in the form of irritability, risky or disruptive behavior, difficulty concentrating, or heightened startle response. Aside from PTSD, many children display a range of subthreshold emotional and behavioral difficulties in response to PTE exposure. Phases of traumatic stress include an acute phase (immediately following the PTE), a peritraumatic phase (first month after the PTE), and a posttraumatic phase (the months following the PTE)—all presenting opportunities for prevention.

Manifestations of traumatic stress vary across development. For example, preschool-aged children may exhibit separation anxiety, temper tantrums, and loss of interest in play activities, whereas school-aged children are more likely to develop social problems, somatization, and feelings of guilt.[7] Adolescents may exhibit social withdrawal, school difficulties, and risky behavior. Childhood exposure to PTEs may cause long-term difficulties lasting into adulthood including heightened risk for mental illness, chronic physical health conditions, worse employment and income outcomes, and interpersonal and social difficulties.[8] Positive family relationships and support may protect youth against negative long-term impacts of trauma,[9] suggesting a potential role of parents and families in prevention and intervention.

CONCEPTUALIZATION FOR PREVENTION OF CHILD TRAUMATIC STRESS

As with most adverse conditions, PTEs can be addressed from a treatment and a prevention perspective. The broad and multifaceted nature of child traumatic stress makes the defining of prevention a more complicated one. The approach adopted here is to break prevention down into 3 categories emphasizing temporal considerations. The first category is the prevention of child exposure to PTEs. Risk for trauma undoubtedly starts with exposure to adverse events or circumstances, some of which might be preventable. This first category focuses only on exposure before it occurs.

The second category is the prevention of child traumatic stress reactions following exposure to the precipitating stressor. The source of the stressor can emanate from inside or outside the family. Extrafamilial PTEs include natural disasters, experiencing or witnessing motor vehicle accidents, witnessing community violence, and childhood bullying. Examples of intrafamilial stressors include child maltreatment, witnessing interparental violence, death of a relative, chronic or life-threatening parental health condition, or parental substance misuse. This category focuses on preventing children's emotional or behavioral difficulties in the short-term aftermath of these adverse events.

The third category is the prevention of negative sequalae following traumatic stress. This category applies to children and youth who have been exposed to PTEs and who have begun to show ill effects. The range of traumatic stressors is broad and can also include scenarios where the exact events or timing are unknown. The preventive interventions in this category focus on mitigating the negative long-term impact of traumatic stress in children exhibiting symptoms.

The Institute of Medicine's prevention framework and stages of health care model is also applicable to prevention of child traumatic stress.[10] In this model, universal prevention focuses on an entire population of children and youth, not just those with specified risks. Selective prevention is aimed at children and youth with identifiable risks and indicated prevention at those beginning to show signs or symptoms of the particular clinical conditions. For prevention of exposure (the first category noted earlier), universal and selective interventions are particularly relevant. Prevention after exposure (the second category) can include universal (all children exposed to the stressful event) or selective (exposed children who belong to a more vulnerable group) interventions. Interventions in the third category, prevention of negative sequalae, would qualify as indicated prevention.

FAMILY-BASED PREVENTIVE INTERVENTIONS AND PROGRAMS

Several behavioral and psychosocial family-based interventions address the prevention or mitigation of child traumatic stress. Focusing on interventions designed to benefit children in the 2- to 15-year-old age range, this article describes several examples of these interventions, which all have in common the central involvement of parents and in some instances whole families. Beyond age range and family involvement, all of the chosen interventions are (1) trauma focused and were specifically designed to address trauma exposure or its consequences; (2) prevention based along the continuum described earlier; and (3) supported by some evidence pertaining to efficacy and feasibility. Most, but not all, of these interventions have been widely disseminated in multiple communities.

PREVENTION OF CHILD EXPOSURE TO POTENTIALLY TRAUMATIC EVENTS

Interventions to prevent child exposure to PTEs draw primarily on universal prevention when focused, for example, on unintentional injuries in the general population. Selective prevention is especially relevant when children are at risk of PTE exposure, such as living in an unsafe neighborhood where there is a heightened risk of community violence exposure or with a parent who uses coercive discipline that may escalate to physical abuse.

ACT Raising Safe Kids Program

The American Psychological Association's Violence Prevention Office (VPO) developed the ACT Program (previously called the Adults and Children Together Against Violence/Parents Raising Safe Kids Program), a group-delivered parenting intervention aimed at the promotion of positive parenting skills to parents and caregivers of children from birth to age 10 years. The program is predicated on the assumption that if parents use physical punishment and other coercive forms of discipline, their children will be more likely to use violence to resolve their own conflicts. The ACT Program, which is part of the VPO's plan to prevent child maltreatment and youth violence, uses an educational format to address ages and stages of child development, parent-child relationships, and positive parenting free from abuse. Multiple studies suggest that the ACT Program yields improvement in self-reported parenting.[11,12] For example, one study that randomized parents to the program versus services as usual found a significant reduction in self-reported harsh parenting despite a significant increase in parenting stress.[11] A multisetting study that randomized parents to intervention and control conditions found gains on self-reported parenting measures, notwithstanding 50% attrition in the recruited sample and failure to use intent-to-treat analysis.[12] The available studies of the ACT Program relied solely on parental self-report of parenting, without providing convergence from other outcome sources such as observation of parent-child interaction or independent measures of child maltreatment. Access to the ACT Program, which is being disseminated in the United States and in other countries, can be found at https://www.act.apa.org.

Triple P—Positive Parenting Program System

The Triple P—Positive Parenting Program (Triple P) is a multilevel system of parenting support interventions designed to promote healthy parenting at the familial and population levels, to reduce child's social-emotional and behavior problems, and to prevent child maltreatment.[13,14] Rather than a single program, Triple P is an array of programs of varying intensities, applications, and formats, all sharing a common set of positive parenting principles, an emphasis on parental and child self-regulation, and a large menu of parenting mini-strategies. Delivery modalities include extended sessions with individual families, brief parental consultation, a group format, large parenting "seminars," and online programs. Triple P has been subjected to considerable research over more than 25 years. The full evidence base, which reflects more than 350 published evaluation studies including 175 randomized controlled trials, can be found at https://pfsc-evidence.psy.uq.edu.au. A consistent outcome across Triple P studies has been demonstrable reduction of coercive parenting practices.[14] With respect to prevention of child maltreatment, a population-level place randomization study showed that counties where Triple P was disseminated through workers in several service sectors reduced substantiated maltreatment cases, foster care placements, and hospital-treated child maltreatment injuries, compared with control counties.[15,16] Access to Triple P, which is being disseminated in the United States and 29 other countries, can be found at https://www.triplep.net/glo-en/home/.

SafeCare

SafeCare is a home-delivered intervention intended primarily for use with parents in the child welfare system who have exhibited substantiated or suspect child abuse or neglect.[17] The program focuses on families with a child aged 0 to 5 years. The program seeks to promote (1) a nurturing relationship, focusing on skills for positive parent-child interactions; (2) a safe environment to protect against neglect and unintentional injury, including childproofing the home; and (3) caregiver skills for child health, to prevent risk factors for medical neglect. The evidence base in support of SafeCare includes several controlled outcome studies.[18–20] The program has produced significant outcomes in terms of reducing child-maltreatment recidivism, increasing parenting skills, decreasing use of violent discipline practices, and improving child functioning. SafeCare, which is available in the United States, Canada, and six other countries, is accessible at https://safecare.publichealth.gsu.edu/about-safecare/.

Prevention of Childhood Unintentional Injuries

The broad area of prevention for childhood unintentional injuries crosses over into family-based programming. Pediatricians and family practice physicians routinely provide guidance to parents regarding, for example, empirically supported strategies to prevent bicycle accidents, swimming accidents[21] and drowning, fires in the home, gun accidents, injury or death from motor vehicle crashes, poisoning, and thermal injuries (eg, scalding).[21,22] Communication of the safe practices in these various contexts can combine public health and primary care mainly in universal prevention.

PREVENTION OF CHILD TRAUMATIC STRESS REACTIONS FOLLOWING EXPOSURE

Following exposure to stressful events, it is possible to intervene within the peritraumatic phase via family-based interventions with the goal of early prevention of traumatic stress reactions. The aim of these programs is to prevent the onset of clinically significant distress.

Disaster Recovery Triple P

Disaster Recovery Triple P (DRTP)[23] is a single-session universal parenting seminar intervention designed to prevent children's traumatic stress reactions following recent (within 1–3 months) exposure to a natural disaster event. DRTP was initially developed in response to the 2010 to 2011 floods in Queensland, Australia, a major natural disaster affecting 2.5 million people. Within the Triple P system described earlier, it is a level 2 "light touch" psychoeducational seminar comprising didactic content, disaster-related media clips, and video-recorded interviews with families affected by disasters. Content includes psychoeducation about the range of children's responses to disasters, common triggers for disaster-related distress, strategies for supporting children and managing media exposure, and parents' self-care. An overarching theme is that although dangerous things happen, the world is not always dangerous. DRTP was implemented with 196 parents following the Queensland floods, and attendees reported high levels of satisfaction with the program and high intentions to implement the parenting advice.[24] A quasi-experimental study with 43 parents revealed reductions in parent-reported child in general and disaster-related behavioral and emotional problems at 2-week and 6-month follow-ups.[24]

Child and Family Traumatic Stress Intervention

The Child and Family Traumatic Stress Intervention (CFTSI),[25] a 5- to 8-session intervention for children aged 7 to 17 years and their caregivers, is designed to be delivered within 30 days of a child's PTE exposure with the goal of preventing traumatic stress reactions. In the initial assessment phase of the CTFSI, parent and child reports of child traumatic stress are assessed separately, and discrepancies are discussed as opportunities for improvement in communication. Treatment emphasizes behavioral skills relevant for the family (eg, related to sleep disturbance, depressive withdrawal, oppositional behavior, intrusive thoughts, anxiety and avoidance, and managing traumatic stress reactions). The program incorporates ongoing symptom monitoring from child and parent perspectives, providing further opportunities to improve communication about the child's functioning. Following treatment completion, the family may be referred for a future booster session or more intensive treatment of PTSD as needed.

In a randomized pilot trial conducted with 112 families in the United States, children who received the CFTSI showed lower posttraumatic stress symptom severity and were 65% less likely to meet diagnostic criteria for PTSD at 3-month follow-up, compared with control children who had received supportive therapy.[25] PTSD symptom clusters of avoidance and reexperiencing, but not hyperarousal symptoms, were significantly reduced in the CFTSI condition. Some evidence has accrued that the CTFSI can reduce caregiver posttraumatic stress[26] and discrepancies between parent and child report of symptoms.[27] The pilot trial was conducted with a racially and ethnically diverse US sample, and intervention materials are available in English and Spanish. More information is available on the program Web site (https://medicine.yale.edu/childstudy/communitypartnerships/cvtc/cftsi/).

FOCUS Family Resilience Program

The Families OverComing Under Stress (FOCUS) Family Resilience Program[28] is designed to improve family functioning and reduce parent and child distress for families who have experienced stressful or traumatic events. Initially designed for military families facing difficulties following deployment, FOCUS is also implemented more broadly in community mental health, medical, and school settings.[28] The program generally applies to children ages 3 years and older, with some adaptations made for preschool-aged children. The program consists of 8 to 12 sessions, initially with parents only, then with children only, and finally with the whole family. Drawn from 3 evidence-based interventions,[29–31] core elements of the intervention include eliciting family concerns and goals, educating the family regarding child development and common reactions to trauma, developing a shared family narrative of the traumatic events, enhancing openness and effective family communication, and developing family resilience skills (eg, emotion regulation, goal setting). The intervention uses a narrative timeline technique in which individual members and the family as a whole construct a visual representation of major events and experienced distress, aimed at reducing misunderstandings contributing to family conflict.

Nonrandomized evaluations with military families have shown that participation in the FOCUS program was associated with reductions in parent and child distress and improvements in child emotional and behavioral adjustment,[32,33] with evidence of family functioning improvement as a mediator.[32] The FOCUS program has been implemented with military and civilian, single- and two-parent household, foster and adoptive, and immigrant families, as well as families experiencing stress related to community violence, chronic illness, domestic violence, parental substance use, and grief.[28] A list of FOCUS sites is available on the Web site (https://focusproject.org/).

Care Process Model for Pediatric Traumatic Stress

The Care Process Model for Pediatric Traumatic Stress (CPM-PTS)[34,35] addresses pediatric traumatic stress for children aged 0 to 18 years within primary care settings through screening and a stratified treatment approach based on symptom severity. Based on the premise that traumatic events are highly prevalent and can lead to negative mental health outcomes, the CPM-PTS relies on screening tools, early identification, and a structured integrated-care approach to prevent ill effects of trauma exposure. Screening tools include the Safe Environment for Every Kid screener[36] for children aged 0 to 5 years and the Pediatric Traumatic Stress Screening Tool[34] for children aged 6 to 18 years. When trauma exposure is identified, traumatic stress is managed by (1) making any necessary reports to child protective services or law enforcement for suspected child maltreatment; (2) responding to suicide risk as needed; and (3) pursuing one level of a stratified array of therapeutic options matched to severity of traumatic stress reaction. The CPM-PTS can be delivered by nonmental health professionals including primary care clinic staff. The CPM-PTS as a universal approach can be implemented with all families in pediatric primary care settings. Outcomes of a pilot trial of CPM-PTS in a US primary care setting are forthcoming. The CPM-PTS can be delivered in English or Spanish and the manual outlines adaptations for special populations (eg, refugees, homeless children).[35] A manual with screening tools, decision trees, and resources for brief intervention may be found at https://utahpips.org/cpm.

PREVENTION OF NEGATIVE SEQUELAE OF TRAUMATIC STRESS

Trauma-exposed youth who experience clinically significant traumatic stress symptoms are at elevated risk for a host of negative long-term outcomes, such as depression and other mental health concerns, substance use disorders, physical health conditions, family problems, and worse economic outcomes in adulthood.[8] For trauma-exposed youth who are already showing clinically significant symptoms of traumatic stress, family-based prevention programs may prevent the negative sequelae and reduce the likelihood of long-term functional impairment.

Trauma-Focused Cognitive Behavioral Therapy

Trauma-Focused Cognitive Behavioral Therapy (TF-CBT)[37] is a family-based intervention targeting traumatic stress in children and adolescents aged 3 to 18 years and their nonoffending caregivers. TF-CBT is designed for youth who have experienced traumatic events and are already demonstrating traumatic stress reactions such as PTSD symptoms, depression, anxiety, and behavioral problems. Typically 8 to 25 sessions in length with a combination of individual child, parent, and conjoint components, intervention content is divided into 3 phases: (1) stabilization (including psychoeducation, cognitive and emotional coping skills, and parenting skills); (2) trauma narrative and processing; and (3) consolidation (including *in vivo* exposure, enhancing parent-child communication about the traumatic event, and preventing future revictimization through safety planning).

TF-CBT has a strong evidence base and is considered a gold-standard treatment of child traumatic stress including PTSD.[38] At least 13 randomized controlled trials have shown the program's efficacy in reducing children's symptoms of PTSD, depression, and behavior problems, compared with attention or waitlist controls or treatment as usual.[38,39] TF-CBT has been implemented and evaluated with families from a wide range of cultural backgrounds, in low- and middle-income countries and other low-resourced settings, with youth affected by commercial sexual exploitation, with youth in foster care, and in several other populations. Cultural adaptations for TF-CBT have been documented for several US (eg, American Indian/Alaska Native, Latinx, Black/African American, refugee) and global (eg, Congolese, Jordanian, Tanzanian, Zambian) populations.[40] TF-CBT is available in many communities, with a database of certified TF-CBT providers found on the program's Web site (https://tfcbt.org/).

Alternatives for Families: A Cognitive Behavioral Therapy

The Alternatives for Families: A Cognitive Behavioral Therapy (AF-CBT)[41] program addresses risk factors and consequences of family conflict, caregiver physical aggression, or child physical abuse. AF-CBT is designed for families with children aged 5 to 17 years where (1) the caregiver engages in physically aggressive discipline, physical abuse, or angry/hostile stance toward the child; (2) the child exhibits externalizing behavior problems and/or trauma-related symptoms, or (3) the family engages in coercive and conflictual interactions. AF-CBT targets factors at (1) the parent level, for example, parental hostility and anger, negative attributions about the child, and ineffective or harsh parenting practices; (2) the child level, for example, child's anger, anxiety, trauma-related distress, social interaction skills, behavioral problems, and negative self-attributions; and (3) the family level, for example, familial coercive or conflicted interactions. Progressing through 3 phases—namely engagement and psychoeducation, individual skill building, and family applications—AF-CBT sessions are conducted depending on topic with either the caregiver alone, child alone, or caregiver and child together. Building on skills training throughout the program, a key component is the "clarification" session, which involves having the caregiver take responsibility for their actions in the abusive or aggressive incidents, recognize and verbalize the impact of the abuse on the child, and plan how to prevent a future incident.

Multiple clinical trials of AF-CBT components reflect the program's effectiveness in reducing parents' use of physically aggressive discipline, parental anger problems and psychological distress, child externalizing behaviors, and family conflict.[41,42] Implementation processes have been evaluated in community mental health and child welfare settings.[43,44] AF-CBT operates in the United States, Canada, and other countries, with program materials available in several languages, and providers are listed on the program's Web site (http://www.afcbt.org/whereisAFCBT).

Combined Parent-Child Cognitive-Behavioral Therapy

Another program to prevent negative sequelae of physical abuse is Combined Parent-Child Cognitive-Behavioral Therapy (CPC-CBT).[45] The program serves families with children ages 3 to 17 years in which there is either substantiated or risk for child physical abuse, although other forms of trauma can be addressed. CPC-CBT aims to help children recover from traumatic stress reactions related to physical abuse or coercive interactions, promote positive and effective parenting, and enhance family safety. Delivered either in an individual family or group format, CPC-CBT typically consists of 16 to 20 sessions comprising 4 phases: engagement, skill building, family safety, and abuse clarification. Early stages of treatment rely more heavily on separate parent and child components, with joint sessions increasing in later stages.

One randomized trial demonstrated that families who received CPC-CBT demonstrated greater improvements in child traumatic stress symptoms and positive parenting compared with those in a parent-only CBT condition.[46] A pilot trial similarly showed pretreatment to posttreatment reductions in parents' use of physical punishment, parental anger, child traumatic stress reactions, and child behavioral problems.[47] Intervention materials are available in English, Spanish, and Swedish, and additional information can be found on the program Web site (https://centers.rowanmedicine.com/cares/services/mentalhealth/cpc-cbt.html).

DISCUSSION

Although child traumatic stress has largely focused on treatment, there is a growing recognition of the need for a cogent public health approach emphasizing prevention.[48] Concentrating only on treatment in the face of a provider shortage in child mental health, exacerbated further by the COVID-19 pandemic, does not reduce or even contain the need for trauma services. A prevention approach is likely to have greater public health impact by (1) reducing the incidence of child trauma exposure, (2) preventing the onset of symptoms for recently trauma-exposed children, and (3) preventing the long-term developmental consequences of traumatic stress. It is valuable to consider opportunities for preventing childhood traumatic stress across multiple time points: before PTE exposure, during the peritraumatic phase, and during the posttraumatic phase after traumatic stress symptoms have begun to appear. The programs described here illustrate ways to reduce the public health burden of child traumatic stress at these different time points.

For children who might experience PTEs, positive family relationships are critical in protecting children from adversity exposure and from the negative short- and long-term outcomes of exposure. Each of the family-based programs discussed here targets aspects of the parent-child relationship using a variety of modalities. Several common strategies characterize many of these programs, including educating parents on common responses to trauma, increasing family communication about the trauma, using exposure-based techniques with the child and family, increasing awareness of safety and the use of safety planning, and reducing parents' coercive discipline strategies and replacing them with positive parenting techniques. Collectively, these programs have shown favorable child, parent, and family outcomes such as less harsh and coercive parenting, improved family functioning, reduced child maltreatment incidence or recidivism, child behavioral and emotional adjustment, fewer child PTSD symptoms, and less caregiver distress. The programs incorporate universal prevention (eg, DRTP, targeting the entire population of parents of disaster-exposed children to prevent negative effects), selective prevention (eg, SafeCare, aimed at families at risk of child maltreatment (re)occurrence), and indicated prevention (eg, TF-CBT, designed for children already exhibiting trauma-related difficulties). Given the shortage of specialty mental health providers for children and the significant barriers to accessing those providers—particularly for youth from underrepresented backgrounds who are disproportionately affected by trauma[3,4]—it is critical to examine other settings and opportunities for the prevention, early identification, and treatment of traumatic stress. Primary care providers such as pediatricians can play a vital role in the effort to address childhood traumatic stress.

SUMMARY

Consistent with a call to embrace a public health, prevention-focused approach to ameliorating the impact of traumatic stress,[48,49] this article described several family-based programs aimed at preventing child traumatic stress, ranging from programs to prevent exposure to PTEs, to those aimed at preventing traumatic stress reactions shortly after exposure, to those preventing the negative long-term consequences of traumatic stress. Programs in these 3 categories draw on universal, selective, and indicated prevention and highlight the importance of parents and families in promoting children's health and addressing children's exposure and reactions to trauma.

CLINICS CARE POINTS

- Pediatric providers should educate caregivers on safety practices to prevent exposure to PTEs.
- To identify traumatic stress early and prevent its negative effects, pediatric providers should consider adopting trauma screening measures in well-child visits across all ages and stages of development.
- Pediatric providers should seek information about potential traumatic stress from multiple sources including both child and caregiver.
- When trauma is identified, pediatric providers should address immediate safety concerns, provide brief education to the family about trauma and common reactions, support parent-child communication about the traumatic event, and teach a relevant coping skill.
- Pediatric providers should familiarize themselves with the family-based prevention programs available locally and provide appropriate encouragement and referrals based on the varying needs of children and families.

ACKNOWLEDGMENTS

The authors would like to acknowledge funding from the National Institute of General Medical Sciences (P20GM130420).

DISCLOSURE

The authors have nothing to disclose.

REFERENCES

1. McLaughlin KA, Koenen KC, Hill ED, et al. Trauma exposure and posttraumatic stress disorder in a national sample of adolescents. J Am Acad Child Adolesc Psychiatry 2013;52(8). https://doi.org/10.1016/j.jaac.2013.05.011.

2. Alisic E, Zalta AK, van Wesel F, et al. Rates of post-traumatic stress disorder in trauma-exposed children and adolescents: Meta-analysis. Br J Psychiatry 2014;204(5):335–40.

3. Roberts AL, Gilman SE, Breslau J, et al. Race/ethnic differences in exposure to traumatic events, development of post-traumatic stress disorder, and treatment-seeking for post-traumatic stress disorder in the United States. Psychol Med 2011;41(1):71–83.

4. Andrews AR, López CM, Snyder A, et al. Polyvictimization, related symptoms, and familial and neighborhood contexts as longitudinal mediators of racial/ethnic disparities in violence exposure across adolescence. J Immigrant Minor Health 2018;0(0):0.

5. Bernard DL, Calhoun CD, Banks DE, et al. Making the "C-ACE" for a culturally-informed adverse childhood experiences framework to understand the pervasive mental health impact of racism on Black youth. J Child Adolesc Trauma 2020;1–15. https://doi.org/10.1007/s40653-020-00319-9.

6. Myers HF, Wyatt GE, Ullman JB, et al. Cumulative burden of lifetime adversities: Trauma and mental health in low-SES African Americans and latino/as. Psychol Trauma Theor Res Pract Policy 2015;7(3):243–51.

7. Goldbeck L, Jensen TK. The diagnostic spectrum of trauma-related disorders in children and adolescents. In: Evidence-Based Treatments for Trauma Related Disorders in Children and Adolescents. ; 2017. doi:10.1007/978-3-319-46138-0_1.

8. Lambert HK, Meza R, Martin P, Fearey E, McLaughlin KA. Childhood trauma as a public health issue. In: Evidence-Based Treatments for Trauma Related Disorders in Children and Adolescents. ; 2017. doi:10.1007/978-3-319-46138-0_3.

9. Goodrum NM, Kilpatrick DG, Smith DW, et al. Longitudinal relations among adolescent risk behavior, family cohesion, violence exposure, and mental health in a national sample. J Abnormal Child Psychol 2020;48(11):1455–69.

10. Please replace the ref#10 with the following details.]National Academies of Sciences, Fostering Healthy Mental, Emotional, and Behavioral Development in Children and Youth: A National Agenda. Washington, DC: The National Academies Press; 2019. https://doi.org/10.17226/25201.

11. Portwood SG, Lambert RG, Abrams LP, et al. An evaluation of the adults and children together (ACT) against violence parents raising safe kids program. J Prim Prev 2011;32(3–4):147–60.

12. Knox M, Burkhart K, Cromly A. Supporting positive parenting in community health centers: The ACT Raising Safe Kids Program. J Community Psychol 2013;41(4):395–407.

13. Sanders MR. Triple P-positive parenting program as a public health approach to strengthening parenting. J Fam Psychol 2008;22(4):506–17.

14. Sanders MR, Mazzucchelli TG, editors. The power of positive parenting: transforming the lives of children, parents, and communities using the Triple P system. New York, NY: Oxford University Press; 2017. Available at: https://www.oxfordclinicalpsych.com/view/10.1093/med-psych/9780190629069.001.0001/med-9780190629069. Accessed December 2, 2021.

15. Prinz RJ, Sanders MR, Shapiro CJ, et al. Population-based prevention of child maltreatment: The U.S. triple P system population trial. Prev Sci 2009;10(1):1–12.

16. Prinz RJ, Sanders MR, Shapiro CJ, et al. Addendum to "Population-Based Prevention of Child Maltreatment: The U.S. Triple P System Population Trial.". Prev Sci 2016;17(3):410–6.

17. Lutzker JR, Edwards A. Safecare: Towards wide-scale implementation of a child maltreatment prevention program. Int J Child Health Hum Development 2009; 2(1):7–15.

18. Chaffin M, Hecht D, Bard D, et al. A statewide trial of the Safecare home-based services model with parents in child protective services. Pediatrics 2012;129(3): 509–15.

19. Whitaker DJ, Self-Brown S, Hayat MJ, et al. Effect of the SafeCare© intervention on parenting outcomes among parents in child welfare systems: A cluster randomized trial. Prev Med 2020;138(November 2019):106167.

20. Guastaferro K, Lutzker JR. A methodological review of SafeCare®. J Child Fam Stud 2019;28(12):3268–85.

21. Jullien S. Prevention of unintentional injuries in children under five years. BMC Pediatr 2021;21:1–11.

22. DeGeorge KC, Neltner CE, Neltner BT. Prevention of unintentional childhood injury. Am Fam Physician 2020;102(7):411–7.

23. Cobham VE, McDermott B, Haslam D, et al. The role of parents, parenting and the family environment in children's post-disaster mental health. Curr Psychiatry Rep 2016;18(6). https://doi.org/10.1007/s11920-016-0691-4.

24. Cobham VE, Mcdermott B, Sanders MR. Parenting support in the context of natural disaster. In: Sanders MR, Mazzucchelli TG, editors. The Power of Positive Parenting: Transforming the Lives of Children, Parents, and Communities Using the Triple P System. Oxford University Press; 2017. p. 272–83.

25. Berkowitz SJ, Stover CS, Marans SR. The child and family traumatic stress intervention: Secondary prevention for youth at risk of developing PTSD. J Child Psychol Psychiatry Allied Disciplines 2011;52(6):676–85.

26. Hahn H, Putnam K, Epstein C, et al. Child and family traumatic stress intervention (CFTSI) reduces parental posttraumatic stress symptoms: A multi-site meta-analysis (MSMA). Child Abuse Neglect 2019;92(April):106–15.

27. Hahn H, Oransky M, Epstein C, et al. Findings of an early intervention to address children's traumatic stress implemented in the child advocacy center setting following sexual abuse. J Child Adolesc Trauma 2016;9(1):55–66.

28. Saltzman WR. The FOCUS family resilience program: an innovative family intervention for trauma and loss. Fam Process 2016;55(4):647–59.

29. Rotheram-Borus MJ, Lee M, Lin YY, et al. Six-year intervention outcomes for adolescent children of parents with the Human Immunodeficiency Virus. Arch Pediatr Adolesc Med 2004;158(8):742–8.

30. Layne CM, Saltzman WR, Poppleton L, et al. Effectiveness of a school-based group psychotherapy program for war-exposed adolescents: a randomized controlled trial. J Am Acad Child Adolesc Psychiatry 2008;47(9):1048–62.

31. Beardslee WR, Wright EJ, Gladstone TRG, et al. Long-term effects from a randomized trial of two public health preventive interventions for parental depression. J Fam Psychol 2007;21(4):703–13.

32. Lester P, Stein JA, Saltzman W, et al. Psychological health of military children: Longitudinal evaluation of a family-centered prevention program to enhance family resilience. Mil Med 2013;178(8):838–45.

33. Lester P, Saltzman WR, Woodward K, et al. Evaluation of a family-centered prevention intervention for military children and families facing wartime deployments. Am J Public Health 2012;102(SUPPL. 1):48–54.

34. Keeshin B, Byrne K, Thorn B, et al. Screening for trauma in pediatric primary care. Curr Psychiatry Rep 2020;20(60). https://doi.org/10.3928/19382359-20200921-01.

35. Keeshin B, Shepard L, Giles L, et al. Diagnosis and management of traumatic stress in pediatric patients: a care process model. 2020. Available at: https://utahpips.org/.

36. Dubowitz H, Feigelman S, Lane W, et al. Pediatric primary care to help prevent child maltreatment: the safe environment for every kid (SEEK) model. Pediatrics 2009;123(3):858–64.

37. Cohen JA, Mannarino AP, Deblinger E. Treating trauma and traumatic grief in children and adolescents. 2nd edition. New York, NY: Guilford Publications; 2017.

38. Dorsey S, McLaughlin KA, Kerns SEU, et al. Evidence base update for psychosocial treatments for children and adolescents exposed to traumatic events. J Clin Child Adolesc Psychol 2017;46(3):303–30.

39. Cohen JA, Deblinger E, Mannarino AP. Trauma-focused cognitive behavioral therapy for children and families. Psychotherapy Res 2018;28(1):47–57.

40. Orengo-aguayo R, Stewart RW, Villalobos BT, et al. Listen, don't tell: partnership and adaptation to implement trauma- focused cognitive behavioral therapy in low-resourced settings 2020;75(8):1158–74.

41. Kolko DJ. Individual cognitive behavioral treatment and family therapy for physically abused children and their offending parents: a comparison of clinical outcomes. Child Maltreat 1996;1(4):322–42.

42. Kolko DJ, Campo Jv, Kelleher K, et al. Improving access to care and clinical outcome for pediatric behavioral problems: a randomized trial of a nurse-administered intervention in primary care NIH Public Access. J Dev Behav Pediatr 2010;31(5):393–404.

43. Kolko DJ, Iselin AMR, Gully KJ. Evaluation of the sustainability and clinical outcome of alternatives for families: a cognitive-behavioral therapy (AF-CBT) in a child protection center. Child Abuse Neglect 2011;35(2):105–16.

44. Kolko DJ, Baumann BL, Herschell AD, et al. Implementation of AF-CBT by community practitioners serving child welfare and mental health: a randomized trial. Child Maltreatment 2012;17(1):32–46.

45. Runyon M, Deblinger E. Combined parent-child cognitive behavioral therapy: an approach to empower families at-risk for child physical abuse; 2013. Accessed December 2, 2021.

46. Runyon MK, Deblinger E, Steer RA. Group cognitive behavioral treatment for parents and children at-risk for physical abuse: an initial study. Child Fam Behav Ther 2010;32(3):196–218.

47. Runyon MK, Deblinger E, Schroeder CM. Pilot evaluation of outcomes of Combined Parent-Child Cognitive-Behavioral Group Therapy for families at risk for child physical abuse. Cogn Behav Pract 2009;16(1):101–18.

48. Magruder KM, Kassam-Adams N, Thoresen S, et al. Prevention and public health approaches to trauma and traumatic stress: a rationale and a call to action. Eur J Psychotraumatology 2016;7. https://doi.org/10.3402/ejpt.v7.29715.

49. Garner A, Yogman M. Preventing childhood toxic stress: Partnering with families and communities to promote relational health. Pediatrics 2021;148(2). https://doi.org/10.1542/peds.2021-052582.

Advances in Supporting Parents in Interventions for Autism Spectrum Disorder

Jessica Bradshaw, PhD[a],*, Katie Wolfe, PhD[b], Robert Hock, PhD[c], Layne Scopano[a]

KEYWORDS

- Autism spectrum disorder • Intervention • Parent-mediated intervention
- Parent training • Social communication • Challenging behavior

KEY POINTS

- Parents and caregivers should be involved in intervention programs for children with autism spectrum disorder (ASD) to improve developmental outcomes and reduce caregiver stress and strain.
- Caregiver-mediated interventions that use naturalistic, developmental, and behavioral approaches are effective for improving social and communication outcomes in infants and children with ASD.
- Strategies for reducing challenging behavior in children with ASD can be effectively taught to caregivers in clinic-, home-, and community-based settings.
- Individualized strategies that support caregivers of children with ASD can reduce burden, strain, and stress, resulting in increased caregiver wellbeing and improved child outcomes.

INTRODUCTION

Recent data suggest that 1 in every 44 children are diagnosed with autism spectrum disorder (ASD).[1] ASD is a highly heterogeneous neurodevelopmental disorder that presents along a spectrum of differences and challenges in social interaction and communication accompanied by restricted interests and repetitive behaviors.[2] Research has shown that early intervention is key in improving the lives and wellbeing of autistic individuals and individuals with ASD.[a] As such, there is an urgent need for the early identification of ASD to accelerate linkage to early intervention services. Routine ASD screenings can take place in pediatrician offices during 18- and

[a] University of South Carolina, 1800 Gervais Street, Columbia, SC 29201, USA; [b] University of South Carolina, 820 Main Street, Columbia, SC 29208, USA; [c] University of South Carolina, 1512 Pendleton Street, Columbia, SC 29208, USA
* Corresponding author.
E-mail address: jbradshaw@sc.edu

Pediatr Clin N Am 69 (2022) 645–656
https://doi.org/10.1016/j.pcl.2022.04.002
0031-3955/22/© 2022 Elsevier Inc. All rights reserved.

24-month well-child visits, followed by referral for further evaluation along with concurrent referral to early intervention. Many early interventions include parents and caregivers as a key component of implementation to increase the child's exposure to intervention strategies as well as the child's generalization of skills. Caregiver involvement in intervention can be considered a caregiver-mediated or caregiver training intervention.[3] Caregiver-mediated interventions refer to those that focus on teaching parents and caregivers how to target core features of ASD, such as social interaction and communication skills. In contrast, caregiver training interventions refer to those that train caregivers on behavioral techniques for decreasing maladaptive behaviors for children with ASD.[3] Largely, this research has focused on the feasibility and acceptability of teaching treatment strategies to caregivers as well as the effectiveness for improving child outcomes. There is an emerging interest in telehealth models for caregiver-implemented interventions as well as caregiver support models for removing barriers to treatment implementation. The focus of this clinical review is to describe recent advances in (1) caregiver-mediated interventions that aim to improve social interaction and communication for children with ASD, (2) caregiver training interventions for reducing challenging behavior, and (3) specific strategies to support caregivers and improve the effectiveness of these interventions.

Supporting Social Interaction and Communication

Social interaction and communication challenges comprise a hallmark feature of ASD. The average age of ASD diagnosis is between 4 and 5 years,[4] yet communication differences can be observed as early as 9 months in infants later diagnosed with ASD.[5] Some of the first social-communication skills to emerge in infancy include shared facial expression and eye gaze, gestures such as showing and giving, and directed vocalizations. Following the onset of first words at around 12 months, additional social-communication skills include coordinating the use of eye contact, gestures, and words as well as combining words to form phrases and sentences. Following the onset of fluent speech and communication, pragmatic language skills, such as conversational turn-taking and context-driven changes in communication style become critical.

Social-communication skills can be supported in infants and children with ASD using naturalistic developmental behavioral interventions (NDBIs). NDBIs are a set of intervention approaches that incorporate the following empirically based components: intervention delivery in natural settings within everyday play- or routine-based contexts, use of activities that are child-preferred and motivating, intervention targets that are informed by developmental science, and intervention strategies based on behavioral principles (eg, antecedent, behavior, consequence).[6] Examples of such NDBIs include Pivotal Response Treatment,[7] the Early Start Denver Model,[8] Early Social Interaction,[9] JASPER,[10] and ImPACT.[11] Caregiver involvement in NDBIs is common practice, but it is especially crucial in the infant and toddler period when play and daily routines are frequently mediated through caregivers.

A surge of interest in caregiver-mediated interventions has occurred over the past decade, and a recent systematic review identified 54 studies of family-mediated interventions that focus on social interaction and communication.[12] The primary goals of these studies were to teach caregivers to implement the intervention with fidelity (ie, deliver the intervention accurately as it was intended) and to improve child skills. To accomplish this, caregivers meet with a trained therapist who teaches the intervention using live modeling, video modeling, role play, and practice with feedback. For example, Project ImPACT[11] is a 24-session manualized caregiver-mediated intervention that targets 4 core social-communication skills: social engagement, language, imitation, and play. During each session, a trained therapist meets with the parent and child to discuss the topic of the day, model intervention strategies with the child, observe the parent practice the strategies with the child, and provide in vivo feedback on intervention implementation. The therapist then provides homework assignments to practice the strategies during daily routines at home. Preliminary results suggest that Project ImPACT significantly increases parent adherence to treatment, improves child social and communication skills, and decreases parent stress and depression.[13] As another example, the parent-mediated JASPER model, is an 8 to 10-week program that teaches parents strategies for improving the frequency of social communication and play acts.[14] Through didactic instruction, therapist modeling, and practice-with-feedback, parents are taught to identify the current play and communication level of their child, follow their child's interests, and insert opportunities for the child to initiate joint attention and engage in joint play routines. Results across multiple studies demonstrate effectiveness in improving joint engagement with a caregiver, responsiveness to joint attention, and diversity of play skills.[14,15] Overall, studies on family-mediated interventions for improving social interaction and communication suggest that these teaching strategies are generally effective in improving caregivers' skills in intervention implementation, resulting in improvements in a variety of child social behaviors, including social engagement, communication skills, and reciprocal social interactions.[12] Some studies also report improvements in parent stress, mental health, and parenting confidence following parent-mediated social-communication interventions.[16,17]

While intervention programs are tailored to the individual skills and motivating activities of each unique child, very little research has been conducted to individualize caregiver-mediated approaches within the unique needs of the caregiver and family context. A recent study showed that parents with high levels of stress before intervention have better outcomes with a lower-intensity intervention, whereas parents with lower stress benefited more from a higher intensity intervention.[18] Parent stress, socioeconomic strain, and autistic traits have also been associated with child outcomes.[19] In general, parents of children with ASD experience heightened levels of stress and mental health challenges[20] and caregiver-implemented interventions result in small, but significant improvements in parenting confidence and, to a lesser degree, mental health.[17] Continuing this emerging line of work will be essential in developing effective and highly tailored coaching strategies.

Telehealth models of caregiver-mediated interventions for social communication are also of particular interest to increase access for rural and lower-resourced families. Synchronous, asynchronous, and hybrid models of remote social-communication NDBIs have been explored, demonstrating the feasibility and preliminary effectiveness for teaching caregivers intervention strategies and improving child social-communication skills, including language, eye contact, and social engagement.[21,22] Some research suggests that telehealth approaches and in-person models result in similar outcomes,[12] while other studies suggest that in-person models are more beneficial.[21]

Interventions for Reducing Challenging Behavior

Challenging behaviors, although not included in the diagnostic criteria for ASD, are common in children and youth with ASD.[23] Current prevalence estimates suggest that 56% to 94% of children with ASD engage in one or more challenging behaviors,[23,24] including aggression, tantrums, self-injury, and property destruction. Challenging behavior can adversely impact the individual's quality of life as well as that of their family, limit access to typical educational and community settings, and increase parental stress. Thus, challenging behavior is a critical treatment target for many individuals with ASD and an area in which caregivers may need significant support.

Researchers have identified numerous empirically supported interventions to address challenging behavior that is rooted in the field of applied behavior analysis (ABA)[25] and an understanding of how events in the environment affect behavior. Specifically, effective intervention begins with identifying the function of challenging behavior, or the conditions under which it is likely to occur. Then, a function-based intervention can be developed with strategies that address the purpose of the behavior.[26] Central to this approach is an emphasis on teaching and reinforcing appropriate behaviors to build adaptive skills and to prevent challenging behavior from reoccurring in the future.[27]

Ample research supports the effectiveness of teaching caregivers of children with ASD to implement interventions for challenging behavior[28,29] and suggests that practice and feedback are integral aspects of effective training because they improve caregivers' implementation fidelity.[30] Unfortunately, the inclusion of practice and feedback in such training can be resource-intensive. Further, therapists who deliver effective caregiver training need specialized knowledge not only about ABA, ASD, and challenging behavior but also about family-centered practice and caregiver coaching.[29] Taken together, these factors can result in reduced access to high-quality caregiver training that maximizes both child and family outcomes.

Recently developed intervention models, including Research Units in Behavioral Intervention (RUBI),[31] Prevent-Teach-Reinforce for Families (PTR),[32] and An Individualized Mental Health Intervention for ASD (AIM HI),[33] focus on scaling up and increasing caregiver access to high-quality training on empirically supported interventions for challenging behavior. Critically, each model includes key ingredients of effective training (ie, caregiver practice and feedback). In addition, each model is manualized and thus can be implemented with consistency by therapists without extensive training in ABA or ASD and who practice in existing service systems such as early intervention and community mental health.

RUBI is a manualized, 16-week caregiver training program for challenging behavior that has been implemented in both individual[31] and group formats.[34] RUBI includes instruction, discussion, modeling, and role play with feedback; caregivers are assigned homework to complete between sessions. Home visits and booster sessions may also be included in the program. Researchers have found that RUBI produces larger decreases in parent-rated child challenging behavior than parent education when implemented individually with families,[3] and that RUBI can be effectively delivered via telehealth to further increase access.[35] Preliminary research also suggests that RUBI is feasible for group delivery in a community-based clinic.[34]

PTR is an intervention model for persistent challenging behavior that incorporates empirically supported strategies and is based on positive behavior support.[27] Positive behavior support is an approach to addressing problem behaviors that focuses on improving the target individual's quality of life by increasing their functional and social skills through evidence-based interventions that fit within the natural environment.[36] Originally developed for school systems, PTR has been adapted[29,37] and manualized for use with families.[32,38] PTR involves a facilitator collaborating with the caregiver to identify the function of specific challenging behavior and develop an individualized function-based intervention that is tailored to the caregiver's preferences, values, and context. The facilitator teaches the caregiver to implement the intervention using modeling, coaching, and feedback. Researchers have served as facilitators in most studies of PTR with families; however, in a notable exception, Rivard and colleagues[39] trained early interventionists to implement PTR with families and reported promising outcomes on parent stress, child challenging behavior, and child-appropriate behavior after the 12-week intervention.

Unlike RUBI and PTR, AIM HI[33] is a therapist training model focused on increasing provider capacity to assist families of children with ASD who engage in challenging behavior. AIM HI is designed to be implemented within ongoing mental health treatment and includes training for therapists in empirically supported interventions for challenging behavior and a manualized protocol to structure sessions with the caregiver and child. Similar to PTR, in AIM HI the therapist and caregiver collaborate to identify the function of the challenging behavior and select function-based intervention strategies. The therapist teaches the caregiver how to implement the intervention strategies during subsequent sessions using modeling, active practice, and feedback. A recent cluster-randomized clinical trial demonstrated significant decreases in the intensity and severity of child challenging behavior[40] and significant increases in parent-reported competence[41] following AIM HI as compared with routine care (ie, typical therapy in the community mental health clinic).

While these models of supporting caregivers can decrease cost and increase access to high-quality training, caregivers may still experience barriers to participation related to therapist capacity and logistics of attending trainings.[42] Families of young children with ASD may access funding for behavioral services and supports through a variety of service systems, including Part C Early Intervention, Medicaid, and private insurance. However, it can be difficult for families to navigate these complex systems and even when they do, they may be placed on a wait list for services due to therapist capacity limitations. In addition, researchers have identified racial, ethnic, and socioeconomic disparities in service use by families who have a child with ASD. Clinicians can support families in accessing services by providing information about available services in a culturally responsive way and by focusing on the coordination of care. Making behavioral supports available in the local community can reduce transportation costs and logistical barriers related to travel, and providing child care during parent training may also increase access for underrepresented groups.[43]

Technology can also be leveraged to reduce some of these barriers. Telehealth can reduce travel time and costs, and it can be as effective as face-to-face training for supporting families in addressing challenging behavior.[44] Asynchronous support, such as online training programs and apps, can make empirically supported interventions more accessible to families and circumvent shortages in providers who are qualified to train families.[42] For example, Barton and colleagues[45] developed the Family Behavior Support App, which prompts caregivers to enter information about their child's challenging behaviors and then uses algorithms to suggest individualized, function-based interventions tailored specifically to the child. The app also includes supplemental training videos to support caregivers' implementation of intervention strategies.

Strategies to Enhance Caregiver Implementation

The aforementioned interventions have strong evidence to support their effectiveness in addressing challenging behaviors and social communication differences in children with ASD. However, the effectiveness of caregiver-implemented interventions depends, in large part, on caregivers' ability to use the skills correctly and consistently in everyday life. This is no small task, given a large amount of time, energy, and expense required to achieve significant child improvements. A recent systematic review found that parent-implemented interventions required parents to participate in training between 2 and 48 hours over periods ranging from 5 weeks to 2 years.[46]

Parents were also asked to devote regular time to implementing the intervention with their child (30 min/d to 20 hours per week).[46] Caregiver-implemented interventions require caregivers to learn new ways of thinking, acting, and communicating with their child. Changing habitual patterns of caregiver–child interaction requires consistent effort and focused attention without an immediate reward as child behavior change often happens over a period of weeks and months. Therefore, caregiver motivation and social-emotional support are vital to success.

Caregiver stress and interventions

A high level of chronic stress can impede intervention implementation because it reduces a caregiver's ability to learn new concepts and skills, regulate their emotions, and stay "tuned-in" to their child.[47,48] Therefore, clinicians are encouraged to assess caregivers' current level of stress and anticipate the potential impact of any proposed intervention. Introducing a new ASD parenting intervention was found to decrease parent stress in some studies and increase stress in other studies.[49] On the one hand, parents gain confidence and parenting efficacy as they receive guidance and learn new skills for helping their child grow. On the other hand, they are learning a number of complex strategies and shifting time and energy away from other family members and responsibilities.[49] Some parents may also experience stress and frustration if the new parenting skills are inconsistent with their parenting style or cultural beliefs about parent–child relationships.[50]

One strategy researchers are using to address parent and caregiver stress is combining caregiver-implemented interventions with stress-reduction interventions. Andrews and colleagues[51] combined Acceptance and Commitment Therapy (ACT) with the RUBI program in an online format and found promising results for parent implementation and child challenging behaviors. ACT is a mindfulness and values-based intervention that reduces parent stress by promoting psychological flexibility and value-consistent action.[52] Weitlauf and colleagues combined Mindfulness-Based Stress Reduction (MBSR) with the parent-implemented Early Start Denver Model (P-ESDM) and found lower parental distress and greater parent mindfulness when compared with parents receiving P-ESDM alone.[53] Hence, evidence to date suggests that adding stress reduction training to parent-mediated ASD interventions successfully reduces stress among parents of children with ASD. It is not yet clear whether such programs improve parenting skill implementation, or whether they can be feasibly delivered in diverse community settings.

Reducing intervention burden

Perception of treatment burden is a predictor of treatment adherence for caregivers of children with ASD.[54] As such, a number of strategies have emerged to reduce the burden of interventions on caregivers and families. Online and telehealth delivery strategies have been developed for several caregiver-implemented interventions for ASD. By leveraging technology, these programs reduce travel time, allow for more flexible scheduling, and reduce the family disruptions that can result from clinic-based and home-based interventions. Perhaps more importantly, they provide access to evidence-based parenting strategies in communities whereby none exist. One systematic review identified several technology-assisted parent-mediated interventions that use diverse delivery formats including: DVD's (animated children's shows and parent training), app-based games and programs, self-paced computer courses with videos and self-quizzes, weekly virtual coaching with a trained clinician, and augmented reality glasses providing real-time emotion feedback to the child.[55] The researchers concluded that these interventions are feasible to deliver and acceptable to parents, but that their effectiveness as standalone interventions has not yet been adequately demonstrated.[55] Other strategies for reducing burden include providing childcare and respite care to assist with other caregiving responsibilities, offering flexible appointment times including nights and weekends, and helping parents strengthen their informal support networks with people who can provide emotional

Table 1
Features of autism spectrum disorder and associated caregiver-implemented intervention strategies

Features of Autism Spectrum Disorder in Childhood	Caregiver-Implemented Intervention Strategies	Intervention Examples
Social Communication and Interaction	*Naturalistic Developmental Behavioral Intervention Strategies for Supporting Social Communication*	*Teaching Social Communication*
Reduced verbal and nonverbal communication of interests, emotions, or affect Limited initiation of social interactions Limited understanding of gestures and body language Difficulty playing with others Reduced or atypical response to social engagement initiated by others	Follow the child's interests and provide opportunities to communicate within natural interactions Reinforce good attempts to communicate Provide opportunities for child to engage in joint play routines	During bath time, if the child reaches for the bubble bath, the caregiver can create an opportunity for the child to request "bubbles." When the child says a good approximation for "bubbles," the caregiver provides natural reinforcement by giving the child bubbles.
Restricted Interests and Repetitive Behaviors	*Function-Based Behavioral Interventions for Reducing Challenging Behavior*	*Reducing Challenging Behavior*
Reduced flexibility with routines and distress in response to small changes Hyper-fixation on certain objects or interests Restricted patterns of play (eg, lining up objects) accompanied by distress to outside interference Hyper- or hyporeactivity to sensory stimuli	Use functional behavior assessment to determine the function (or cause) of the challenging behavior Prevention or antecedent strategies include modifying the environment or increasing the predictability of a routine. Instructional strategies include teaching replacement behaviors and improving adaptive behavior skills Consequence strategies include differentially reinforcing adaptive behaviors	For a child who has difficulty transitioning between activities, a caregiver can use a visual schedule and visual timer to increase predictability and prepare for transitions. For a child who demonstrates challenging behavior when wanting an activity to stop, a caregiver can teach appropriate communication (eg, an approximation of "I need a break"), prompt for this communication at the onset or right before the challenging behavior, and reinforce attempts to communicate by providing a break.

Note: Features of ASD based on diagnostic criteria from the DSM-5.[1]

and practical support (eg, other parents of children with ASD, extended family, neighbors, friends, church).

One of the most powerful and often overlooked sources of support for parents is other family members. Most caregiver-mediated interventions are conducted with the primary caregiver alone.[49] This places additional responsibility on the primary caregiver to educate and obtain buy-in from other caregiving adults and child siblings. Additionally, the effectiveness of the intervention can be dampened if family members, particularly coparents, undermine intervention strategies when they are with the child. Conversely, coparent support and coordination are associated with increased parenting efficacy and reduced stress among parents of children with ASD.[56] For these reasons, clinicians are encouraged to educate all family members about the purpose and process of the intervention and why it will work. Including family members in the intervention process whenever possible reduces the burden on the primary caregiver to be the "champion" of the intervention. Research has shown that including other caregivers and siblings during intervention delivery improves parent–child, sibling, and marital relationships.

DISCUSSION

Best care practices for children with ASD involve caregivers in intervention implementation (for a summary, **Table 1**). Interventions that adopt naturalistic, developmental, and behavioral approaches are effective for improving some of the hallmark features of ASD—social interaction and communication. Studies of caregiver-mediated NDBIs have proven their effectiveness while also identifying barriers to treatment implementation, including caregiver strain, stress, and mental health challenges.

Challenging behavior can be a significant stressor for individuals with ASD, caregivers, and the family system. Behavioral strategies that start with identifying the function of the challenging behavior are extremely effective but can require a high degree of expertise and detailed data collection. Caregiver training programs can teach caregivers how to identify functions of behavior and select specific treatment strategies that reduce challenging behaviors. Research shows that caregiver training can be effectively delivered at differing intensities in a variety of settings (eg, home, clinic, community). Access to such training is expanding with technology-based synchronous and asynchronous programs and phone-based apps.

Despite significant progress in caregiver-implemented interventions, substantial barriers to implementation remain. These include parenting stress and strain, caregiver mental health challenges, and accessibility, particularly in rural and lower-resourced communities. In recognition of these barriers, studies that focus on supporting caregivers, independent from child-focused interventions, are emerging. Direct integration of caregiver support strategies into intervention programs is a promising avenue for improving the overall well-being of families affected by ASD.[49]

SUMMARY

Caregivers have become integral to intervention programs for infants and children with ASD and a range of evidence-based, caregiver-implemented interventions have been developed to reduce challenging behaviors and improve social communication. Interventions vary in complexity, mode of delivery, time commitment, and amount of family involvement. While caregivers should not be the sole source of intervention for children with ASD, their ability to incorporate treatment strategies throughout daily routines and activities can enhance developmental outcomes, reduce challenging behavior, and improve their sense of competence and efficacy.

Barriers to treatment implementation exist for caregivers, especially those who are lower resourced and experience high levels of stress and strain. Research on optimal ways to support caregivers is still emerging, but promising strategies include telehealth modes of delivery, coparenting support, and mindfulness-based stress reduction programs. Thus, physicians should consider a family's resources, availability, motivation, and level of stress to recommend interventions in which families are most likely to succeed.

CLINICS CARE POINTS

- Naturalistic, developmental, and behavioral interventions are among the most empirically validated, caregiver-mediated treatments for improving social-communication skills in infants and children with ASD.
- Caregiver training models that use principles of ABA and focus on the development of function-based interventions are effective for reducing challenging behaviors in children with ASD.
- Caregivers of young children with ASD may access training and supports through Part C Early Intervention, Early Childhood Special Education, or ABA therapy funded by Medicaid or private insurance.
- Caregiver-implemented interventions are generally effective for improving parenting confidence, enhancing self-efficacy, and reducing caregiving stress and strain.
- Emerging research suggests that telehealth approaches to caregiver-implemented interventions are effective, but in-person models may be more beneficial for some.
- Strategies for supporting caregivers of children with ASD can include mindfulness-based stress reduction programs, tailored interventions for unique family contexts, and matching intervention approaches and dosage to parent stress levels and available resources.

DISCLOSURE

National Institute of Mental Health (NIMH) K23MH120476National Institute of Child Health and Development (NICHD) R01HD099295 Carolina Autism and Neurodevelopment Research Center Pilot Award.

REFERENCES

1. Maenner MJ, Shaw KA, Bakian Av, et al. Prevalence and Characteristics of Autism Spectrum Disorder Among Children Aged 8 Years — Autism and Developmental Disabilities Monitoring Network, 11 Sites, United States, 2018. MMWR Surveill Summ 2021;70(11):1–16.
2. American Psychiatric Association. Diagnositic and Statistical manual of mental disorders. 5th edition; 2013.
3. Bearss K, Burrell TL, Stewart L, et al. Parent Training in Autism Spectrum Disorder: What's in a Name? Clin Child Fam Psychol Rev 2015;18(2):170–82.
4. Baio J, Wiggins L, Christensen DL, et al. Prevalence of Autism Spectrum Disorder Among Children Aged 8 Years - Autism and Developmental Disabilities Monitoring Network, 11 Sites, United States, 2014. Morbidity mortality weekly Rep Surveill Summ 2018;67(6):1–23.
5. Bradshaw J, McCracken C, Pileggi M, et al. Early social communication development in infants with autism spectrum disorder. Child Development 2021;92(6):2224–34.

6. Schreibman L, Dawson G, Stahmer AC, et al. Naturalistic Developmental Behavioral Interventions: Empirically Validated Treatments for Autism Spectrum Disorder. J autism Dev Disord 2015;45(8):2411–28.

7. Koegel LK, Ashbaugh K, Koegel RL. Pivotal response treatment. In: Lang R, Hancock T, Singh N, editors. Early intervention for young children with autism spectrum disorder. Springer; 2016. p. 85–112.

8. Rogers S, Dawson G. Early start Denver model for young children with autism: promoting language, learning, and engagement. The Guildord Press; 2009.

9. Wetherby AM, Guthrie W, Woods J, et al. Parent-Implemented Social Intervention for Toddlers With Autism: An RCT. Pediatrics 2014;134(6):1084–93.

10. Kasari C, Freeman S, Paparella T. Joint attention and symbolic play in young children with autism: a randomized controlled intervention study. J Child Psychol Psychiatry 2006;47(6):611–20.

11. Ingersoll B, Dvortcsak A. Teaching social communication to children with autism: a Practicioner's Guide to parent training. The Guilford Press; 2010.

12. Pacia C, Holloway J, Gunning C, et al. A Systematic Review of Family-Mediated Social Communication Interventions for Young Children with Autism. Rev J Autism Dev Disord 2021. https://doi.org/10.1007/s40489-021-00249-8.

13. Stadnick NA, Stahmer A, Brookman-Frazee L. Preliminary Effectiveness of Project ImPACT: A Parent-Mediated Intervention for Children with Autism Spectrum Disorder Delivered in a Community Program. J Autism Developmental Disord 2015; 45(7):2092–104.

14. Kasari C, Gulsrud AC, Wong C, et al. Randomized Controlled Caregiver Mediated Joint Engagement Intervention for Toddlers with Autism. J Autism Developmental Disord 2010;40(9):1045–56.

15. Kasari C, Dean M, Kretzmann M, et al. Children with autism spectrum disorder and social skills groups at school: a randomized trial comparing intervention approach and peer composition. J Child Psychol Psychiatry 2016;57(2):171–9.

16. Manohar H, Kandasamy P, Chandrasekaran V, et al. Brief Parent-Mediated Intervention for Children with Autism Spectrum Disorder: A Feasibility Study from South India. J Autism Developmental Disord 2019;49(8):3146–58.

17. MacKenzie KT, Eack SM. Interventions to Improve Outcomes for Parents of Children with Autism Spectrum Disorder: A Meta-Analysis. J Autism Developmental Disord 2021. https://doi.org/10.1007/s10803-021-05164-9.

18. Estes A, Yoder P, McEachin J, et al. The effect of early autism intervention on parental sense of efficacy in a randomized trial depends on the initial level of parent stress. Autism : Int J Res Pract 2021;25(7):1924–34.

19. Shalev RA, Lavine C, di Martino A. A Systematic Review of the Role of Parent Characteristics in Parent-Mediated Interventions for Children with Autism Spectrum Disorder. J Developmental Phys Disabilities 2020;32(1):1–21.

20. Padden C, James JE. Stress among Parents of Children with and without Autism Spectrum Disorder: A Comparison Involving Physiological Indicators and Parent Self-Reports. J Dev Phys disabilities 2017;29(4):567–86.

21. McGarry E, Vernon T, Baktha A. Brief Report: A Pilot Online Pivotal Response Treatment Training Program for Parents of Toddlers with Autism Spectrum Disorder. J Autism Developmental Disord 2020;50(9):3424–31.

22. Ingersoll B, Wainer AL, Berger NI, et al. Comparison of a Self-Directed and Therapist-Assisted Telehealth Parent-Mediated Intervention for Children with ASD: A Pilot RCT. J Autism Developmental Disord 2016;46(7):2275–84.

23. Kanne SM, Mazurek MO. Aggression in Children and Adolescents with ASD: Prevalence and Risk Factors. J Autism Developmental Disord 2011;41(7):926–37.

24. McTiernan A, Leader G, Healy O, et al. Analysis of risk factors and early predictors of challenging behavior for children with autism spectrum disorder. Res Autism Spectr Disord 2011;5(3):1215–22.
25. Hume K, Steinbrenner JR, Odom SL, et al. Evidence-Based Practices for Children, Youth, and Young Adults with Autism: Third Generation Review. J Autism Developmental Disord 2021;51(11):4013–32.
26. Dunlap G, Kern L. Perspectives on Functional (Behavioral) Assessment. Behav Disord 2018;43(2):316–21.
27. Carr JE, Sidener TM. On the relation between applied behavior analysis and positive behavioral support. Behav Analyst 2002;25(2):245–53.
28. Fettig A, Barton EE. Parent Implementation of Function-Based Intervention to Reduce Children's Challenging Behavior. Top Early Child Spec Education 2014;34(1):49–61.
29. Sears KM, Blair KSC, Iovannone R, et al. Using the Prevent-Teach-Reinforce Model with Families of Young Children with ASD. J Autism Developmental Disord 2013;43(5):1005–16.
30. Wyatt Kaminski J, Valle LA, Filene JH, et al. A Meta-analytic Review of Components Associated with Parent Training Program Effectiveness. J Abnorm Child Psychol 2008;36(4):567–89.
31. Bearss K, Johnson C, Handen B, et al. A Pilot Study of Parent Training in Young Children with Autism Spectrum Disorders and Disruptive Behavior. J Autism Developmental Disord 2013;43(4):829–40.
32. Dunlap G, Strain P, Lee J, et al. Prevent-teach-reinforce for families. Brookes; 2017.
33. Brookman-Frazee L, Baker-Ericzén M, Stadnick N, et al. Parent Perspectives on Community Mental Health Services for Children with Autism Spectrum Disorders. J Child Fam Stud 2012;21(4):533–44.
34. Edwards GS, Zlomke KR, Greathouse AD. RUBI parent training as a group intervention for children with autism: A community pilot study. Res Autism Spectr Disord 2019;66:101409. https://doi.org/10.1016/j.rasd.2019.101409.
35. Bearss K, Burrell TL, Challa SA, et al. Feasibility of Parent Training via Telehealth for Children with Autism Spectrum Disorder and Disruptive Behavior: A Demonstration Pilot. J Autism Developmental Disord 2018;48(4):1020–30.
36. Kincaid D, Dunlap G, Kern L, et al. Positive behavior support: A proposal for updating and refining the definition. J Positive Behav Interventions 2016;18(2):69–73.
37. Argumedes M, Lanovaz MJ, Larivée S, et al. Using the Prevent-Teach-Reinforce model to reduce challenging behaviors in children with autism spectrum disorder in home settings: A feasibility study. Res Autism Spectr Disord 2021;86:101804. https://doi.org/10.1016/j.rasd.2021.101804.
38. Joseph HM, Farmer C, Kipp H, et al. Attendance and Engagement in Parent Training Predict Child Behavioral Outcomes in Children Pharmacologically Treated for Attention-Deficit/Hyperactivity Disorder and Severe Aggression. J Child Adolesc Psychopharmacol 2019;29(2):90–9.
39. Rivard M, Mello C, Mestari Z, et al. Using Prevent Teach Reinforce for Young Children to Manage Challenging Behaviors in Public Specialized Early Intervention Services for Autism. J Autism Developmental Disord 2021;51(11):3970–88.
40. Brookman-Frazee L, Roesch S, Chlebowski C, et al. Effectiveness of Training Therapists to Deliver An Individualized Mental Health Intervention for Children With ASD in Publicly Funded Mental Health Services. JAMA Psychiatry 2019;76(6):574.

41. Brookman-Frazee L, Stadnick NA, Lind T, et al. Therapist-Observer Concordance in Ratings of EBP Strategy Delivery: Challenges and Targeted Directions in Pursuing Pragmatic Measurement in Children's Mental Health Services. Adm Policy Ment Health Ment Health Serv Res 2021;48(1):155–70.

42. Raulston TJ, Hieneman M, Caraway N, et al. Enablers of Behavioral Parent Training for Families of Children with Autism Spectrum Disorder. J Child Fam Stud 2019;28(3):693–703.

43. Smith KA, Gehricke JG, Iadarola S, et al. Disparities in service use among children with autism: A systematic review. Pediatrics 2020;145(Supplement_1): S35–46.

44. Lindgren S, Wacker D, Suess A, et al. Telehealth and Autism: Treating Challenging Behavior at Lower Cost. Pediatrics 2016;137(Supplement_2):S167–75.

45. Barton EE, Meadan H, Fettig A. FSBApp.

46. Trembath D, Gurm M, Scheerer NE, et al. Systematic review of factors that may influence the outcomes and generalizability of parent-mediated interventions for young children with autism spectrum disorder. Autism Res 2019;12(9): 1304–21.

47. Sanders MR, Turner KMT, Metzler CW. Applying Self-Regulation Principles in the Delivery of Parenting Interventions. Clin Child Fam Psychol Rev 2019;22(1): 24–42.

48. Rovane AK, Hock RM, January SAA. Adherence to behavioral treatments and parent stress in families of children with ASD. Res Autism Spectr Disord 2020; 77:101609. https://doi.org/10.1016/j.rasd.2020.101609.

49. Factor RS, Ollendick TH, Cooper LD, et al. All in the Family: A Systematic Review of the Effect of Caregiver-Administered Autism Spectrum Disorder Interventions on Family Functioning and Relationships. Clin Child Fam Psychol Rev 2019; 22(4):433–57.

50. Lord C, Charman T, Havdahl A, et al. The Lancet Commission on the future of care and clinical research in autism. Lancet 2021. https://doi.org/10.1016/S0140-6736(21)01541-5.

51. Andrews ML, Garcia YA, Catagnus RM, et al. Effects of Acceptance and Commitment Training Plus Behavior Parent Training on Parental Implementation of Autism Treatment. Psychol Rec 2021. https://doi.org/10.1007/s40732-021-00496-5.

52. Hayes SOC, Luoma JB, Bond FW, et al. Acceptance and commitment therapy: Model, processes and outcomes. Behav Res Ther 2006;44(1):1–25.

53. Weitlauf AS, Broderick N, Stainbrook JA, et al. Mindfulness-Based Stress Reduction for Parents Implementing Early Intervention for Autism: An RCT. Pediatrics 2020;145(Supplement_1):S81–92.

54. Hock R, Kinsman A, Ortaglia A. Examining treatment adherence among parents of children with autism spectrum disorder. Disabil Health J 2015;8(3):407–13.

55. Pi HJ, Kallapiran K, Munivenkatappa S, et al. Meta-Analysis of RCTs of Technology-Assisted Parent-Mediated Interventions for Children with ASD. J Autism Developmental Disord 2021. https://doi.org/10.1007/s10803-021-05206-2.

56. May C, Fletcher R, Dempsey I, et al. Modeling Relations among Coparenting Quality, Autism-Specific Parenting Self-Efficacy, and Parenting Stress in Mothers and Fathers of Children with ASD. Parenting 2015;15(2):119–33.

The Importance of Addressing Multilevel Transactional Influences of Childhood Obesity to Inform Future Health Behavior Interventions

Dawn K. Wilson, PhD[a,*], Nicole Zarrett, PhD[a],
Allison M. Sweeney, PhD[b]

KEYWORDS

- Obesity prevention • Child health • Risk factors • Multi-level interventions

KEY POINTS

- Although past research has identified numerous factors related to obesity, such factors are typically evaluated in isolation, which provides a limited understanding of how these factors work together across systems.
- This article synthesizes past research on childhood obesity into a coherent model of the etiology of obesity to support a broader conceptual basis for understanding the etiology of obesity and to inform future health behavior interventions.
- We provide an overview of the multi-level, transactional influences on childhood obesity by reviewing recent research on genetic, biological, cognitive, sociocultural, social determinants, and intrapersonal regulatory processes.
- We highlight the usefulness of using a theoretic framework that includes the ecological model to identify the mechanisms that may reinforce social nurturance and the promotion of positive social environments across contexts.
- Finally, we provide a series of examples of multi-level transactional interventions for improving childhood weight-related behaviors and outcomes, including interventions that intervene within community, school, and health care settings.

Across the past 2 decades, the emergence and persistence of worldwide obesity have led to numerous empirical studies on understanding the origins of childhood obesity and other related health outcomes. The prevalence of obesity increases from

[a] Department of Psychology, Barnwell College, University of South Carolina, Columbia, SC 29208, USA; [b] College of Nursing, University of South Carolina, 1601 Greene Street, Columbia, SC 29208, USA
* Corresponding author.
E-mail address: wilsondk@mailbox.sc.edu

Pediatr Clin N Am 69 (2022) 657–669
https://doi.org/10.1016/j.pcl.2022.04.003
0031-3955/22/© 2022 Elsevier Inc. All rights reserved.

childhood through adolescence, ranging from 13.9% of children ages 2 to 5, to 18.4% of children ages 6 to 11, and 20.6% of adolescents ages 12 to 19.[1] Approximately 80% of adolescents with obesity continue to have obesity in adulthood,[2] which increases the risk for health complications across the lifespan, including cardiovascular disease, type 2 diabetes, cancer, and premature death.[3–5] Such findings highlight the critical need to understand the causes and correlates of obesity to better identify and develop effective interventions to prevent obesity.

A growing evidence-base demonstrates the independent contributions of several obesity-related person- and context-level factors. These factors range from genetic, biological, cognitive, and sociocultural factors. More specifically, these factors include stress-related life events, family processes, peer processes, and characteristics and climate of community/neighborhood, school, and home-related risk and protective factors. However, research has largely focused on these factors in isolation, without taking into consideration the other key influences within this developmental system, resulting in a loose array of diverse predictors of obesity without an understanding of how these factors operate together. This article aims to synthesize findings into a coherent model of the etiology of obesity to support a broader conceptual basis for understanding the etiology of obesity and to inform future health behavior interventions.

The emergence of obesity-related health behaviors and outcomes may be conceptualized using a transactional biopsychosocial ecological developmental model.[6,7] Drawing from Relational and Dynamic Systems life course perspectives of human development[8,9] and Bioecological/Ecological Models of health behavior specifically[9,10] this model highlights the dynamic interactions between individuals (ie, biological, intrapersonal characteristics) and their environments over time to promote and optimize health, but also postulates directional and temporal sequence and key transactions between key components of the developmental system. This model posits that biological factors and sociocultural contexts (eg, poverty) place certain children at greater risk in early life than others, but life experiences (eg, social determinants including parenting, peers, neighborhood, school) function to moderate and/or mediate this level of risk. That is, reciprocal coactions between biological/genetic characteristics, contexts, and life experiences lead to recursive iterations across time that exacerbates or diminish an individual's level of risk for developing obesity and comorbidities (**Fig. 1**).

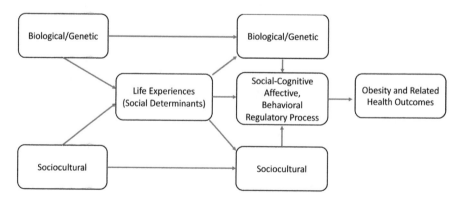

Fig. 1. Transactional biopsychosocial echological developmental model of the etiology of obesity.

As depicted in **Fig. 1**, early biological/genetic characteristics and sociocultural factors directly influence health-related life experiences, and in a transactional way, these life experiences, in turn, influence the development and later expression of biological and genetic characteristics (ie, reinforce or alter epigenetic processes) and sociocultural factors (eg, access to health care). Together, transactions that occur over time between biological/genetic and sociocultural factors with life experiences shape children's health-related social-cognitive, affective, and behavioral regulatory processes and consequent health outcomes. The role of the health care providers in promoting positive social environments across contexts to reduce childhood obesity has become of increasing interest in health promotion. Although in isolation, only a small proportion of reductions in long-term morbidity is explained by access to health care.[11] Thus, models are needed to integrate the health care sector into broader community-based trials, which we highlight through our focus on ecological systems as a framework.

Health is not predetermined but is actively construed through the choices and actions that individuals' take within the range of resources and constraints of their biological and contextual situations across time. Thus, social, cognitive, affective, and behavioral regulatory/motivational processes within the child are proposed to mediate the relation between life experiences and health outcomes. Key characteristics of the individual including health-based self-concepts and identities, self-efficacy, and expectancies for the future achievement of one's health-based goals, as well as one's interest/value of health promotive or compromising behaviors have been identified as primary predictors of individuals' engagement in health behaviors.[12–14] These intrapersonal processes are highly influenced by biological/genetic factors, contexts, and life experiences and thus, typically support continuity of risk pathways. However, they can also function as protective factors and are common mechanisms targeted in behavioral interventions to mitigate risk.[15–18] Example studies cover a vast range of health-promoting behaviors including dietary modifications through fostering youth self-efficacy for healthy eating,[17,19,20] building efficacy for engaging in physical activity[21] and fostering efficacy through key change agents to impact physical activity and wellbeing within youth settings.[16,18,22]

In this model, there is no single causal agent for obesity, but rather obesity results from multiple diverse risk and promotive factors. The various potential relations between these diverse factors indicate that there are numerous pathways that may link to obesity, and thus, that there are likely multiple different obesity etiology subtypes, each with its own unique developmental pathway. Across the past decade, research adopting a biopsychosocial[23] or relational systems perspective[8,9] that considers multiple systems of influence across development has uncovered some important transactions between biological and sociocultural factors, social determinants, and intrapersonal processes to inform critical points of intervention during the developmental years.

BIOLOGICAL, SOCIOCULTURAL, SOCIAL DETERMINANTS, AND INTRAPERSONAL REGULATORY PROCESSES

Health is a process that develops over the lifespan with the prenatal through adolescent years viewed as a critical time in the lifespan for the acquisition and optimization of health capacities that set the course for health through adulthood. These are particularly formidable years in which individuals are highly dependent on the degree of access they have to external environmental resources to establish and maintain optimal health functioning.[9,24] Therefore, under optimal developmental conditions, this early part of the lifespan through adolescence can be used to invest in future health potentials and build health "reserves" to help offset the impact of declines experienced in later life.[24]

Within this framework, obesity pathways are conceived as driven by cumulative risk or protective processes with the development of earlier health promotion/compromising behaviors influencing one's capacity for later health and wellbeing. Risk for obesity begins before conception with a woman's access to resources/health habits and reproductive health (eg, nutrition, neural-hormonal environment) and continues postconception with transactions between maternal prenatal health and resources and fetal and postnatal development.[25] Specifically, past research has shown that biological and sociocultural factors including mother's weight status before pregnancy, gestational weight gain, nutritional constraint/undereating during pregnancy, and an infant's birth weight, as well as early postnatal life experiences of overnutrition/overfeeding are strongly associated with risk of developing obesity later in childhood.[26] Increasing evidence suggests that father's health and wellbeing are also important for fetal, infant, and childhood health with paternal depression, anxiety, and stress shown to influence prenatal development indirectly through the impact it has on maternal stress and experiences during pregnancy,[27,28] and may make significant and unique direct contributions to infant's postpartum physiologic regulatory functioning independent to the impact of maternal stress and wellbeing.[29,30] Thus, biological and life experiences alter epigenetic processes within the fetus/infant that lead to long-term changes in metabolism (eg, through genes that impact lipid, carbohydrate metabolism, appetite-energy balance, insulin resistance, inflammatory response),[26] shape affective, social-cognitive, and behavioral processes around eating (eg, food preferences, eating schedules) and physical activity, all of which can further reinforce parental health promotion and feeding practices and perpetuate risk for obesity in a transactional way.

Likewise, sociocultural influences such as poverty, food insecurity, racial discrimination, lack of neighborhood resources, have been shown to impact parental stress which prompts similar effects on fetal and postfetal epigenetic processes and development (ie, low birth weight) and cascading transactional processes on intrapersonal factors and risk for obesity.[31,32] Such findings highlight the importance of addressing access and quality of women's health care (pregestational, prenatal, postnatal care) and for developing interventions to support positive parenting and to reduce parental stress including consideration for the broader environmental and social factors that drive chronic stress (eg, discrimination, poverty). There is a growing interest in addressing the stress and coping of underserved communities to reduce obesity-related risk in early childhood.[33]

These early prenatal/postnatal developmental experiences that either support or hinder the development of personal capacity (ie, physical, social, cognitive assets) continue to cumulate through the childhood and adolescent years and determine the degree to which individuals are capable of effectively interacting with their biological, physical, and social environments to optimize their health trajectories and to adapt to any unanticipated or expected challenges. Similarly, early disruptions in capacity development can set in motion a cascade of developmental processes that result in an individual's reduced capacity to optimize their health potential. However, life experiences and the exposure and degree of influence of key social determinants change as youth develop, offering opportunities for youth to "change course" in terms of their personal capacity to optimize health and offset risk for obesity. For example, during infancy through childhood, individuals have the greatest dependency on parents and other caregivers and thus risks and promotive factors embedded within the family system are likely to have the greatest influence on health.[34]

Furthermore, previous research has demonstrated that an authoritative (autonomy-supportive) parenting style that supports attachment, warmth, and the development of self-regulation skills, as well as positive parental feeding practices (eg, parental monitoring of diet) and physical activity practices (eg, role modeling, values) are highly influential on children's physical activity and dietary intake.[17,35,36] At the other extreme, exposure to adverse experiences, such as violence or maltreatment, or day-to-day impoverished interactions between parent and child due to parent depression, economic hardship, and/or stress during is associated with lifelong health risk behaviors and outcomes including obesity, heart disease, and type 2 diabetes.[34,37,38] However, the influence of other social systems (ie, school policies, teachers, peers, and daycare/aftercare) can play a role in supporting youth health behaviors, values, and regulatory processes. These processes operate to reinforce positive transactions within the home context that support health capacity and mitigate risk for obesity by forming new types of transactions between youth and biological, sociocultural, and life experiences.

As youth develop through adolescence, their increased orientation toward and interactions with peers also function to exacerbate the impact of social and cultural systems on youths' health behaviors.[39,40] Previous research has demonstrated the powerful influence that adolescents' peers and friends have on their health promotive[41] and risky behaviors[42] through a variety of mechanisms including direct modeling effects and normative influences. However, transactions between peer experiences and other key social systems, like family are whereby there is the greatest influence. For example, in a diverse middle school sample of youth[43] investigators found significant interactions between peer social functioning and familism (support/connections from family) whereby the positive effect of peer social functioning on healthy eating was greater for those youth who reported higher (vs lower) familism. Peer influences have also been shown to interact with other key social systems and life experiences to either reinforce existing transactional processes or set in motion new transactional processes. For instance, neighborhood socioeconomic deprivation has been shown to be significantly associated with higher fat mass and increased likelihood of overweight/obesity among adolescents. These relations hold even after accounting for youth key health behaviors (ie, physical activity, sedentary behavior, diet quality, demographics),[44] indicating that health behaviors do not fully explain the relations between neighborhood deprivation and weight status.

In summary, theoretic, and empirical research support the importance of taking a future-orientated approach to health promotion that addresses biological, sociocultural, contextual, and intrapersonal risk and protective factors and their cumulative, and transactional, impact on youths' health trajectories.

THEORETIC FRAMEWORKS FOR MULTI-LEVEL TRANSACTIONAL INTERVENTIONS

The transactional biopsychosocial ecological approach emphasizes the importance of addressing the transactional relationship between individuals and their environments over time.[23] This framework advocates for multi-level interventions that address individual-level characteristics (eg, behavioral skills, coping strategies), social-environmental factors (eg, social groups, cultural influences), *and* broader community and environmental factors (eg, policy, neighborhood access), as the most effective approach for promoting health behavior change,.[10,45]

Aligned with biopsychosocial ecological theories,[8,10] we also propose that to effectively increase health-promoting behaviors it is important to understand the mechanisms that may reinforce social nurturance and the promotion of positive social environments across contexts.[46] Growing evidence suggests that interventions that integrate family systems, motivational, and behavioral theories are likely to have greater success in producing positive health behavior changes.[20,46,47] Family Systems Theory (FST) emphasizes the importance of parental nurturance and monitoring to promote shared-decision making as youth transition into young adulthood.[20,48] Consistent with FST, Self-Determination Theory (SDT) also emphasizes the importance of the social environment for promoting an individual's long-term motivation for health behavior change, including the need for autonomy, competency, and relatedness across a variety of social contexts. These include interactions with health care providers, family, and friends.[13,49] Social Cognitive Theory (SCT) proposes that the self-regulation of health behaviors is shaped, in part, by broader social and structural impediments to change, including impediments rooted in the inequitable delivery of health services.[12,15] Thus, we argue for a transactional biopsychosocial ecological model[6,7] that integrates elements from FST,[48] SDT,[13] and SCT[12,15] to better understand how individual-level behavioral skills and autonomous motivation, family-level support, and communication, as well as other key socializing agents and contexts (eg, health care, school, peers), are shaped by and help shape later biological characteristics and influence how youth interact with the broader social environment and life experiences, to facilitate health.

Many past studies have not been successful, and we argue, through the examples provided later in discussion, for more multilevel (systems) approaches to address the broad range of influences on the development and prevention of early childhood obesity.

EXAMPLES OF HEALTH BEHAVIOR INTERVENTIONS THAT INTEGRATE COMMUNITY COMPONENTS

An example of a community-based multi-level intervention is the 'B'More Healthy Communities for Kids' study, a cluster-randomized controlled trial that aimed to prevent obesity among youth ages 9 to 15 years by improving household purchasing of healthy food and dietary intake.[50] The intervention targeted multiple systems, including individual, interpersonal, environmental, and policy-related changes. Community "zones" consisting of a recreation center in a low-income predominantly African American neighborhood in the Baltimore area were randomized to the multi-component environmental intervention or served as a comparison. The intervention involved partnerships between recreation centers and local corner stores and/or carryout restaurants within walking distance. The recreation centers implemented a peer-led nutrition educational program targeting healthier beverages, snacks, and cooking methods. Complementing this approach, the corner stores were incentivized to stock and promote healthier food items, and social media was used to engage caregivers (eg, sharing recipes, advertising upcoming events). Caregivers also received text messages with information about goal-setting strategies and tips for implementing healthy eating strategies. City stakeholders were encouraged to support policies to sustain a healthy community food environment.[51]

At the end of the 5-year trial, youth in the intervention significantly increased their purchasing of healthier foods and beverages, with this effect being more pronounced among younger adolescents.[52] Among older adolescents, there was a significant reduction in the percentage of calories from sweet snacks and desserts. This trial highlights the value of intervening within community settings, addressing the community food environment, and engaging both adolescents, caregivers, and stakeholders through a range of individual, interpersonal and environmental strategies.

Another example of a multi-level intervention is "Shape Up Summerville," a community-based participatory study that tested whether an environmental intervention could prevent obesity among early elementary school children.[53,54] In a 2-year trial, 3 socio-demographically matched communities participated, with 2 acting as controls and one receiving the environmental intervention. The environmental intervention was designed to promote enhanced opportunities for physical activity and healthy eating by intervening across multiple systems and contexts, including targeting changes at school, at home, and through broader community initiatives/policies. Intervention activities included a walk to school program, increased access to healthy foods in school cafeterias, delivery of an after-school curriculum targeting greater physical activity and healthy snacks, parent outreach and education, partnering with local restaurants to promote healthy menus, and the development of community-based policies to promote long-term sustainability (eg, wellness programs, pedestrian safety). Multiple groups and organizations within the community were involved in the delivery of the intervention, including children, parents, teachers, before and after-school staff, school food-service providers, policy makers, health care providers, restaurants, and local media.

After 1 year of intervention delivery, children in the intervention community demonstrated a greater decrease in their body mass index (BMI) z-score than those in the control communities,[53] which was sustained through 2-year follow-up.[54] Additionally, the intervention resulted in a significant reduction in sugar-sweetened beverage consumption, increased participation in sports and physical activity, and reduced screen time.[55] The positive impact of the intervention also extended to parents, as demonstrated by a significant decrease in parent BMI.[56] Taken together, the results from the Shape Up Summerville support the efficacy of intervening across multiple systems to promote the behavioral and environmental changes to prevent childhood obesity.

EXAMPLES OF HEALTH BEHAVIOR INTERVENTIONS THAT INTEGRATE HEALTHCARE COMPONENTS

One example of a multi-level intervention with a health care component is the Stanford GOALS study, a randomized controlled trial that tested the efficacy of a multi-component intervention relative to a health education program for reducing BMI among overweight/obese children (ages 7–11) from low socioeconomic status neighborhoods.[52] The multi-component intervention included a community-based after school sports program, a home-based behavioral counseling family component to promote healthy eating, reduce screen time, and behavioral counseling from a primary care provider. The study sample was primarily Latinx and thus the intervention was also culturally tailored to address cultural values, such as collectivism, familism, and religiosity. The multi-component intervention targeted a variety of processes, including individual factors (eg, behavioral skills training), interpersonal factors (eg, social belongingness, team sports), and environmental factors (eg, changes to the home environment).

Over the course of the 3-year study, children in the intervention gained less weight in the first 2 years of the intervention than those in the health education comparison group, but this effect was not sustained in 3 years.[52] Similar positive intervention effects were observed in the first 2 years of the program for physical activity, diet changes, and cardiometabolic risk factors. Although the overall retention rate was high, there was steady drop off in participation over time, which may explain why the treatment effect was not maintained. While the Stanford GOALS study was successful at promoting behavioral change across a 2-year period, these findings highlight some of the challenges of engaging families long-term and the need to better understand how to best capitalize on partnerships across community and health care settings to promote maintaining healthy body weight.

Another example of a multi-level intervention with a primary care component is the "Now Everybody Together for Amazing and Healthful Kids" (NET-WORKS), a randomized trial that integrated home, community, primary care, and neighborhood intervention strategies to prevent obesity among preschool-age children.[57] Participants were recruited through primary care clinics, with the intervention being implemented across multiple settings, including brief counseling component delivered in pediatric primary care settings, a home-based program, community-based parenting classes and linking families to neighborhood and community resources for physical activity and healthy eating. The home-based program targeted positive parenting strategies, goal-setting, and home-based environmental changes to promote positive changes in healthy eating, physical activity, and screen time. The parenting classes were designed to build on the curriculum from the home-based program, while also providing an opportunity for enhanced social support. Additionally, primary care providers received updates from the home-based program on families' progress and delivered key messages to parents during their child's annual checkup visit.

Compared with usual care, children in the NET-WORKS intervention demonstrated significantly lower energy intake and television watching at 24 and 36 months. However, these behavioral changes do not seem to have facilitated significant changes in BMI as a change in BMI was not significantly different between the intervention and usual care at 24 or 26 months. Secondary analyses revealed that children who had overweight or obesity at baseline showed a greater decrease in BMI in the intervention than usual care at 36 months. Additionally, the intervention seems to have been more effective for Hispanic children (58.4% of the total sample) who demonstrated a lower BMI in the intervention at 36 months. The NET-WORKS study provides an example of how partnerships with health care providers can be used to facilitate recruitment and the reinforcement of key intervention elements. These results suggest that future multi-level interventions may benefit from tailoring toward baseline weight status and differences across racial and ethnic groups.

Another example of a multi-component intervention in a primary care setting is a trial by Resnicow and colleagues,[53] which targeted parents of overweight/obese children ages 2 to 8 years. This trial targeted health care providers and parents as 2 key ecological systems critical to obesity prevention. Pediatric offices were randomized to deliver 1 of 3 interventions: usual care; motivational interviewing sessions delivered by a primary care provider; or motivational interviewing sessions delivered by a primary care provider plus additional sessions delivered by a registered dietician (RD). Integrating elements from SDT,[13] motivational interviewing is a counseling style that promotes autonomous motivation and self-initiated behavioral change through techniques such as shared decision-making and reflective listening.[54] Additionally, integrating elements from SCT,[15] the motivational interviewing sessions included behavioral skills training to facilitate positive changes in diet and physical activity among families, included goal setting, self-monitoring, and problem solving. At the 2-year follow-up, youth whose parent received motivational interviewing and behavioral skills training from both a primary care provider and an RD had a significantly lower BMI than the usual care group. These results suggest that families may benefit most from nurturing environments that integrate autonomy support and behavioral skills training from multiple sources.

In another primary care setting obesity treatment trial, the "High Five for Kids" study,[55] children (ages of 2–6 years) were randomized to an integrated health care provider plus family systems approach versus a usual care comparison. Primary caregivers were randomized to an SDT and SCT weight loss program or a usual care program. Ten pediatric facilities participated to test whether a family-based intervention delivered in a primary care setting would be successful in reducing BMI and obesity-related behaviors, such as television watching, and fast-food consumption among overweight/obese children. Health care providers at the pediatric offices were trained to integrate multiple medical care providers (nurse practitioners, physicians, medical assistants). The intervention specifically integrated motivational interviewing and targeted behavioral skills for promoting weight loss, including decreasing television viewing, and intake of fast food and sugar-sweetened beverages over 1 year.

After 1 year, there was no significant difference in BMI; however, the researchers found there was a significant reduction in the amount of time children viewed television in the intervention group relative to the usual care group.[56] Importantly, only half of the families completed 2 of the 6 sessions. In a post hoc analysis, the researchers found a significant change in BMI among girls, but not boys. This study highlights that although the intervention that integrated SDT and SCT had a positive impact on obesity-related health behaviors, future studies may need to consider further strategies for maximizing participant engagement and intervention dose through addressing broader social contextual factors beyond the health care setting. Specifically, while the above studies suggest that a multi-systems approach that integrates multiple practitioners and families into the interventions are critical for obesity prevention in young children, future studies should consider engaging broader community systems to reinforce long-term changes.

SUMMARY AND RECOMMENDATIONS

In this article, we advocate for a biopsychosocial ecological approach to health for understanding the early risk of obesity in youth that integrates a multi-level systems approach. We argue that positive health is actively construed through the choices and actions that youth take within the range of resources and constraints of their biological and contextual situations across time. Obesity pathways are conceived as driven by cumulative risk or protective processes with the development of earlier health promotion/compromising behaviors influencing one's capacity for later health and wellbeing. Risk for obesity begins before conception with access to resources/ health habits and reproductive health (eg, nutrition, neural-hormonal environment) and continues postconception with transactions between paternal prenatal health and resources and fetal and postnatal development.[25] A critical focus is on the role of protective factors in early childhood through early adulthood that we argue comes from a broad range of social contextual factors including family, peers, teachers, and health care providers.

We provided examples of theoretic approaches to weight management and weight loss that integrate multi-level systems which demonstrated the efficacy and effectiveness of multi-level intervention approaches that engage youth, family, communities, and health care providers. While these studies begin to provide evidence of impact of addressing multiple systems including health care providers, families, and communities, the causal determinants of change are not well understood. Future research is needed to further address the mediators and mechanisms through which this transactional model can be used for the early prevention of childhood obesity. Further research will provide the evidence base to develop a comprehensive approach for developing policies to address early childhood social and environmental risk factors for obesity at a national level.

CLINICS CARE POINTS

- Health behavior interventions for treating childhood obesity show that it is important to include multiple systems including health care providers, families, peers, and community engagement to effectively improve health behaviors and weight loss in youth.

- While community-based trials have begun to integrate primary care sectors into their obesity prevention and treatment approaches for effective childhood weight loss, further efforts are needed to better understand long-term compliance.

- Family systems factors such as parental nurturance, monitoring, and role modeling are critical to address given these early childhood factors place children are greater risk or protection of developing obesity.

- Increasing evidence suggests that creating a positive social and supportive environment and integrating behavioral skills such as goal setting are critical intervention components across all systems for early childhood obesity prevention.

DISCLOSURE

All authors have nothing to disclose.

REFERENCES

1. Hales CM, Carroll MD, Fryar CD, et al. Prevalence of Obesity Among Adults and Youth: United States, 2015-2016. NCHS Data Brief 2017;(288):1–8.
2. Simmonds M, Llewellyn A, Owen CG, et al. Predicting adult obesity from childhood obesity: a systematic review and meta-analysis. Obes Rev 2016;17(2): 95–107.
3. Reilly JJ, Kelly J. Long-term impact of overweight and obesity in childhood and adolescence on morbidity and premature mortality in adulthood: systematic review. Int J Obes 2011;35(7):891–8.
4. Franks PW, Hanson RL, Knowler WC, et al. Childhood Obesity, Other Cardiovascular Risk Factors, and Premature Death. N Engl J Med 2010;362:485–93.
5. Kelsey MM, Zaepfel A, Bjornstad P, et al. Age-related consequences of childhood obesity. Gerontology 2014;60:222–8.
6. Cicchetti D, Toth SL, Maughan A. An Ecological-Transactional Model of Child Maltreatment. In: Sameroff A, Lewis M, editors. Handbook of developmental Psychopathology. 2nd edition. Kluwer Academic/Plenum Press; 2000. p. 689–722.
7. Sameroff A, Chandler M. Reproductive risk and the continuum of care-taking casualty. In: Horowitz F, editor. Review of child development research. Chicago: University of Chicago Press; 1975. p. 187–244.
8. Bronfenbrenner U. Making human beings human: Bioecological perspectives on human development. Thousand Oaks, CA: Sage Publications; 2005.
9. Halfon N, Larson K, Lu M, et al. Russ S. Lifecourse health development: Past, present and future. Matern Child Health J 2014;18(2):344–65.
10. Sallis J, Owen N, Fisher E. Ecological models of health behavior. In: Glanz K, Rimer BK, Viswanath K, editors. Health behavior: theory, research, and practice. 5th edition. San Fransisco, CA: John Wiley & Sons; 2015. p. 43–64.
11. Kaplan R. More than medicine: the Broken Promise of American health. Cambridge, MA: Harvard University Press; 2019.
12. Bandura A. Social Foundations of Thought and action: a social cognitive theory. New Jersey: Prentice-Hall, Inc; 1986.

13. Ryan RM, Deci EL. Self-determination theory and the facilitation of intrinsic motivation, social development, and well-being. Am Psychol 2000;55:68–78.
14. Eccles JS, Wigfield A. Motivational Beliefs, Values, and Goals. Annu Rev Psychol 2002;53(1):109–32.
15. Bandura A. Health Promotion by Social Cognitive Means. Health Educ Behav 2004;31(2):143–64.
16. Zarrett N, Law LH, Wilson DK. Connect through PLAY: A randomized controlled feasibility trial in after school programs to increase youth physical activity. J Behav Med 2021;44:379–91.
17. Wilson DK, Sweeney AM, Van Horn ML, et al. The Results of the Families Improving Together (FIT) for Weight Loss Randomized Trial in Overweight African American Adolescents. Ann Behav Med 2022. https://doi.org/10.1093/abm/kaab110.
18. Zarrett N, Wilson DK, Sweeney A, et al. An overview of the Connect through PLAY trial to increase physical activity in underserved adolescents. Contemp Clin Trials 2022;114:106677.
19. Bestle SMS, Christensen BJ, Trolle E, et al. Reducing Young Schoolchildren's Intake of Sugar-Rich Food and Drinks: Study Protocol and Intervention Design for "Are You Too Sweet?" A Multicomponent 3.5-Month Cluster Randomised Family-Based Intervention Study. Int J Environ Res Public Health 2020;17(24):9580.
20. Wilson DK, Kitzman-ulrich H, Resnicow K, et al. An Overview of the Families Improving Together (FIT) for Weight Loss Randomized Controlled Trial in African American Families. Contemp Clin Trials 2016;42:145–57.
21. Olander EK, Fletcher H, Williams S, et al. What are the most effective techniques in changing obese individuals' physical activity self-efficacy and behaviour: a systematic review and meta-analysis. Int J Behav Nutr Phys Act 2013;10(1):29.
22. Toledano-González A, Labajos-Manzanares T, Romero-Ayuso D. Well-Being, Self-Efficacy and Independence in older adults: A Randomized Trial of Occupational Therapy. Arch Gerontol Geriatr 2019;83:277–84.
23. Adler RH. Engel's biopsychosocial model is still relevant today. J Psychosom Res 2009;67(6):607–11.
24. Li S-C, Freund AM. Advances in Lifespan Psychology: A Focus on Biocultural and Personal Influences. Res Hum Dev 2005;2(1–2):1–23.
25. Larqué E, Labayen I, Flodmark CE, et al. From conception to infancy — early risk factors for childhood obesity. Nat Rev Endocrinol 2019;15(8):456–78.
26. Lillycrop KA, Burdge GC. Epigenetic changes in early life and future risk of obesity. Int J Obes 2011;35(1):72–83.
27. Tanner Stapleton LR, Schetter CD, Westling E, et al. Perceived partner support in pregnancy predicts lower maternal and infant distress. J Fam Psychol 2012;26(3):453–63.
28. Vismara L, Rollè L, Agostini F, et al. Perinatal parenting stress, anxiety, and depression outcomes in first-time mothers and fathers: A 3-to 6-months post-partum follow-up study. Front Psychol 2016;7:938.
29. Gao M, Brown MA, Neff D, et al. Prenatal paternal stress predicts infant parasympathetic functioning above and beyond maternal prenatal stress. J Reprod Infant Psychol 2021. https://doi.org/10.1080/02646838.2021.1941822.
30. Van Den Berg MP, Van Der Ende J, Crijnen AAM, et al. Paternal depressive symptoms during pregnancy are related to excessive infant crying. Pediatrics 2009;124(1):e96–103.

31. Cao-Lei L, Dancause KN, Elgbeili G, et al. DNA methylation mediates the impact of exposure to prenatal maternal stress on BMI and central adiposity in children at age 13 1/2 years: Project Ice Storm. Epigenetics 2015;10(8):749–61.

32. Dunkel Schetter C, Lobel M. Pregnancy and birth outcomes: a multilevel analysis of prenatal maternal stress and birth weight. In: Baum T, Revenson T, Singer J, editors. Handbook of health psychology, vol. 431-463. London: Psychology Press; 2012. p. 431–63.

33. Quattlebaum M, Kipp C, K WD, et al. A Qualitative Study of Stress and Coping to Inform the LEADS Health Promotion Trial for Overweight African American Adolescents. Nutrients 2021;13:1–18.

34. Repetti RL, Taylor SE, Seeman TE. Risky families: Family social environments and the mental and physical health of offspring. Psychol Bull 2002;128(2):330–66.

35. Loncar H, Wilson DK, Sweeney AM, et al. Associations of parenting factors and weight related outcomes in African American adolescents with overweight and obesity. J Behav Med 2021;44:541–50.

36. Wilson DK, Sweeney AM, Quattlebaum M, et al. The Moderating Effects of the Families Improving Together (FIT) for Weight Loss Intervention and Parenting Factors on Family Mealtime in Overweight and Obese African American Adolescents. Nutrients 2021;13:1745.

37. Amemiya A, Fujiwara T, Shirai K, et al. Association between adverse childhood experiences and adult diseases in older adults: A comparative cross-sectional study in Japan and Finland. BMJ Open 2019;9(8):e024609.

38. Hughes K, Bellis MA, Hardcastle KA, et al. The effect of multiple adverse childhood experiences on health: a systematic review and meta-analysis. Lancet Public Heal 2017;2(8):e356–66.

39. Brown BB, Larson J. Peer relationships in adolescence. In: Lerner RM, Steinberg L, editors. Handbook of adolescent psychology. Hoboken, NJ: John Wiley & Sons, Inc; 2009. p. 74–103.

40. Steinberg L. Cognitive and affective development in adolescence. Trends Cogn Sci 2005;9(2):69–74.

41. Springer AE, Kelder SH, Hoelscher DM. Social support, physical activity and sedentary behavior among 6th-grade girls: A cross-sectional study. Int J Behav Nutr Phys Act 2006;3(1):8.

42. Defoe IN, Semon Dubas J, Romer D. Heightened Adolescent Risk-Taking? Insights From Lab Studies on Age Differences in Decision-Making. Policy Insights Behav Brain Sci 2019;6(1):56–63.

43. Salvy SJ, Miles JNV, Shih RA, et al. Neighborhood, Family and Peer-Level Predictors of Obesity-Related Health Behaviors Among Young Adolescents. J Pediatr Psychol 2017;42(2):153–61.

44. Clennin M, Brown A, Lian M, et al. Neighborhood Socioeconomic Deprivation Associated with Fat Mass and Weight Status in Youth. Int J Environ Res Public Health 2020;17(17):6421.

45. Bronfenbrenner U. Ecological systems theory. In: Vasta R, editor. Six theories of child development: revised formulations and current issues. London: Jessica Kingsley Publishers.; 1992. p. 187–249.

46. Wilson DK, Sweeney AM, Kitzman-Ulrich H, et al. Promoting Social Nurturance and Positive Social Environments to Reduce Obesity in High-Risk Youth. Clin Child Fam Psychol Rev 2017;20:64–77.

47. Kitzman-Ulrich H, Wilson DK, St George SM, et al. The integration of a family systems approach for understanding youth obesity, physical activity, and dietary programs. Clin Child Fam Psychol Rev 2010;13(3):231–53.

48. Broderick CB. Understanding family process: basics of family systems theory. Thousand Oaks, CA: Sage Publications, Inc; 1993.
49. Ng JYY, Ntoumanis N, Thøgersen-Ntoumani C, et al. Self-Determination Theory Applied to Health Contexts. Perspect Psychol Sci 2012;7(4):325–40.
50. Schwendler T, Shipley C, Budd N, et al. Development and Implementation: B'More Healthy Communities for Kid's Store and Wholesaler Intervention. Health Promot Pract 2017;18(6):822–32.
51. Nam CS, Ross A, Ruggiero C, et al. Process Evaluation and Lessons Learned From Engaging Local Policymakers in the B'More Healthy Communities for Kids Trial. Health Educ Behav 2019;46(1):15–23.
52. Trude ACB, Surkan PJ, Cheskin LJ, et al. A multilevel, multicomponent childhood obesity prevention group-randomized controlled trial improves healthier food purchasing and reduces sweet-snack consumption among low-income African-American youth. Nutr J 2018;17(1):1–15.
53. Economos CD, Hyatt RR, Goldberg JP, et al. A community intervention reduces BMI z-score in children: Shape up somerville first year results. Obesity 2007; 15(5):1325–36.
54. Economos CD, Hyatt RR, Must A, et al. Shape Up Somerville two-year results: A community-based environmental change intervention sustains weight reduction in children. Prev Med (Baltim) 2013;57(4):322–7.
55. Folta SC, Kuder JF, Goldberg JP, et al. Changes in diet and physical activity resulting from the shape up Somerville community intervention. BMC Pediatr 2013; 13(1):1–9.
56. Coffield E, Nihiser AJ, Sherry B, et al. Shape up somerville: Change in parent body mass indexes during a child-targeted, community-based environmental change intervention. Am J Public Health 2015;105(2):e83–9.
57. Sherwood NE, French SA, Veblen-Mortenson S, et al. NET-Works: Linking families, communities and primary care to prevent obesity in preschool-age children. Contemp Clin Trials 2013;36(2):544–54.

Seasonal Shifts in Children's Sedentary Behaviors, Physical Activity, and Sleep
A Systematic Review and meta-Analysis

R. Glenn Weaver, PhD*, Caroline Hensing,
Bridget Armstrong, PhD, Elizabeth L. Adams, PhD,
Michael Beets, PhD

KEYWORDS

- Obesity • 24-h movement • Screen time • Pediatric • Sedentary

KEY POINTS

- Movement behaviors like sedentary behaviors, physical activity, and sleep are related to obesity risk for children and may vary throughout the year due to weather, daylight, and climate.
- Movement behaviors may also vary due to the fluctuation of children's exposure to the structure throughout the year (eg, presence or absence of the school day), but past reviews exploring the seasonal fluctuation in children's movement behaviors have failed to account for structure.
- Findings from this review indicate that children are least active during the summer when children are not in school, and winter.
- However, these findings are preliminary because many studies were unclear about when measures were conducted (eg, unclear if measures were conducted when children were on vacation from school or on weekdays, weekend days, or both).
- There is a paucity of data on seasonal variation in sleep indicating a need for further research in this area.

INTRODUCTION

The movement behaviors of children, which include sleep, sedentary behavior, and all levels of physical activity intensity, are related to health outcomes, including obesity.[1] Children's engagement in movement behaviors varies by season for a variety of reasons including, weather patterns (ie, temperature changes, increased/decreased

Arnold School of Public Health, University of South Carolina, Columbia, SC, USA
* Corresponding author. Department of Exercise Science, Arnold School of Public Health, University of South Carolina, Discovery Building, 921 Assembly Street, Columbia, SC 29201.
E-mail address: weaverrg@mailbox.sc.edu

Pediatr Clin N Am 69 (2022) 671–693
https://doi.org/10.1016/j.pcl.2022.04.005
0031-3955/22/Published by Elsevier Inc.

precipitation) and photoperiod (ie, length of daylight). While the season is not a modifiable predictor of children's movement behaviors it is critical to understand how children's movement behaviors shift in relation to season to better design and deliver interventions. For example, understanding when children's movement behaviors are less optimal can optimize intervention timing by informing which season(s) of the year an intervention would most likely result in improved behaviors, while saving costs and resources by not targeting other season(s) of the year when children already engage in healthier levels of movement behaviors.

Previous systematic reviews have established that children's physical activity and sedentary behaviors fluctuate based on season and weather,[2-5] with summer consistently found to be the most physically active month and winter the least active.[3-5] However, no reviews have explored seasonal changes in children's sleep behaviors. Further, past reviews are limited because they have not meta-analytically combined studies to estimate the effect of season.[2-5] Additionally, previous systematic reviews are limited because they have combined physical activity and sedentary data from adults and children, thus precluding the ability to understand the unique patterns of children's health behaviors across seasons due to child-specific factors.[3] Further, previous systematic reviews of the effect of season on children's movement behaviors were conducted nearly a decade ago,[4,5] before an increased consideration of the importance of behaviors along the movement continuum (ie, sleep to vigorous physical activity) and improvements in behavioral measures. Thus, an updated review that includes recent studies is warranted.

A major limitation of past reviews is the failure to account for the presence or absence of the school day during measurement periods, as the structure of a child's day is emerging as a major contributor to children's movement behaviors.[6] The structured days hypothesis posits that the structure of a child's day, defined as preplanned, segmented, and adult-supervised compulsory environments (like a school day), promotes engagement in more healthful behaviors (eg, reduced sedentary, increased physical activity and sleep). This can prevent children's engagement in unhealthy levels of movement behaviors and, in turn, excessive body mass index (BMI) gain. Thus, seasonal variation in children's movement behaviors may be confounded by the presence of a school day in one season (eg, spring) and the absence of a school day during another season (eg, summer).

The purpose of this systematic review and meta-analysis was to examine seasonal shifts in children's movement behaviors while accounting for the presence or absence of structure during the summer.

METHODS

This systematic review was guided and reported in accordance with the Preferred Reporting Items for Systematic reviews and Meta-analyses checklist.[7,8]

Eligibility Criteria

Studies that were repeated cross-sectional or longitudinal were eligible for inclusion if they reported physical activity and/or sleep of children (5–12 years) during 2 or more meteorologic seasons. Baseline and/or control group data from intervention studies was also included as long as it met all other inclusion criteria. Meteorologic seasons were defined as: spring (March 1st–May 31st), summer (June 1st–August 31st), fall (September 1st–November 30th), and winter (December 1st–February 28th). For studies conducted south of the equator meteorological seasons were reversed: fall (March 1st–May 31st), winter (June 1st–August 31st), spring (September 1st–November 30th), and summer (December 1st–February 28th). English language, peer-reviewed published studies were included in the review and no restrictions were placed on the year of publication. Studies were excluded if they only included participants outside of the 5 to 12-year range (ie, younger or older children or adults, unless the study presented data for categorized groups inclusive of ages 5–12); did not report seasonal differences between outcomes; they were intervention studies not including baseline data; and if they selected children because they had a specific health condition (eg, cancer, diabetes) or were part of a select group (eg, elite athletes). Case reports, letters to the editor, conference abstracts, theses or dissertations, and viewpoint articles were excluded.

Information Sources and Search Strategy

A total of 4 electronic databases (PubMed, PsycInfo, Web of Science, and Embase) were searched for relevant studies in September and October of 2020. Search terms in 3 categories; (i) season term (eg, fall), (ii) age group (eg, child), and (iii) outcome (eg, physical activity) were combined using Boolean operators and searched systematically in each database. Titles and abstracts were identified using Medical Subject Heading terms (MeSH-terms) in PubMed. A full list of search terms and an example search strategy for PubMed are included in Supplementary Table 1. When the search strategy identified a systematic review and/or meta-analysis, the references were reviewed for relevant articles.

Data Management and Selection Process

The resulting citations of each search in all databases were downloaded as RIS or XML files and imported into Endnote citation management software (Endnote x9, Clarivate, London, United Kingdom). Duplicates were removed using the Endnote remove duplicate function. Citations were then uploaded into Covidence (Covidence.org, Melbourne, Australia), an online systematic review management software, for screening and review. Titles and abstracts were screened by 2 coauthors (CH & CL) independently to identify those that potentially met inclusion criteria. PDFs for the studies identified for inclusion in the title and abstract screening were then retrieved and reviewed by the same 2 coauthors that completed the title and abstract screening (CH & CL). Where disagreements occurred in both title/abstract and full-text screenings, the first author (RGW) reviewed the disputed article and made the final decision on inclusion.

Data Collection Process

Data extraction on the articles that were passed through the full-text screening was conducted by 2 coauthors (CH & CL). Data were input into a custom extraction spreadsheet created for this review in Microsoft Excel. An author (CL) emailed the corresponding author for articles that did not fully report data to be extracted up to 3 times with a request to provide the missing data.

Data Items

Characteristics extracted from all studies included the following variables: study author, publication year, number of participants, number of female participants, country for which the study was conducted, World Bank Region for which the study was conducted, study design, outcomes measured (physical activity, sedentary behavior, and/or sleep), seasons and months for which the outcomes were measured, if the measure was objective (eg, pedometer, accelerometer) or self-reported, and the mean age of the sample along with a standard deviation when provided. To account for increased structure that might or might not exist during a child's day, 2 pieces of information were extracted. First, data on if measures were collected on weekdays, weekends, or both, and second if the measures included school vacation days. Extraction was customized for each sleep and physical activity/sedentary behavior outcome. For sleep, outcomes included sleep duration (eg, total sleep time), sleep onset, and sleep offset, and sleep other (ie, parent reported if child sleeps more and is tired). Physical activity and sedentary behavior outcomes included sedentary, light physical activity (LPA), moderate physical activity (MPA), vigorous physical activity (VPA), moderate-to-vigorous physical activity (MVPA), steps, and other physical activity outcomes (eg, number of sports enrolled, active transport [eg, walking or biking to school], activity counts). Point estimates (eg, mean, median) and variability of those estimates (eg, standard deviation, standard error, interquartile range, 95% confidence interval) were extracted for each outcome during each season that it was reported. All point estimates were converted to means and all variability estimates were converted to standard deviations according to guidelines from the Cochrane Handbook for Systematic Reviews of Interventions.[9]

Quality Assessment

Two coauthors (CH & CL) examined the risk of bias for each included study independently using relevant metrics on the National Institutes of Health Quality Assessment Tool for Observational Cohort and Cross-sectional Studies.[10] Studies were examined for quality using 10 items. Each item was rated as meeting, not meeting, or cannot determine. Each item rated as meeting was given a score of 1 and items were summed for each study providing an overall risk of bias score.

Data Analysis

The key characteristics of the included studies were tabulated. Standardized mean difference (SMD) effect sizes were calculated for each study across all outcomes in Comprehensive Meta-Analysis (v.3.0). Effect sizes were standardized to account for differences in the direction of scales so that a negative effect consistently meant that a health behavior was worse during the comparison season and a positive effect indicated that a health behavior was better during the comparison season. Meta-analyses were conducted in Stata (v.16.1, StataCorp, College Station, Texas). Because no single season was included in all studies, a multi-step process was undertaken to compare effects between seasons. First, because spring was the most common season measured, spring was compared with fall, summer, and winter. Second, fall was then compared with summer and winter as fall was the second most measured season. Third, winter was then compared with summer. Following the primary analysis, and to account for structure when exploring seasonal changes in behaviors, subanalyses were completed for studies that conducted measures on weekdays and weekends and presented outcomes separately. Subanalyses were also completed for studies that conducted measures while children were attending school and while children were on vacation from school. Vacation subanalyses were only possible for vacation days during the summer as only one study identified that measures were taken on vacation days during a different season.[11] Because multiple effects were nested within study, the robumeta command in Stata was used to calculate 95% confidence intervals around point estimates from robust standard errors.[12] All models included study latitude, sample size, participant age, and use of an objective versus self-report measure of the outcome as covariates. Due to the fact that we intended to generalize the findings beyond the included studies and the meta-analysis included more than 5 studies,[13] all models were conducted using random-effects weighting schemes. To be included in the meta-analyses a comparison between seasons had to be made in 2 or more studies for the outcome in question.[14] The

Benjamini–Hochberg procedure with a false discovery rate of 5% was used to account for multiple comparisons.[15] The I^2 statistical was calculated to evaluate the heterogeneity of estimates for each outcome. Values of 25%, 50%, and 75% were considered to represent low, moderate or high heterogeneity, respectively.[9]

RESULTS
Prisma Flow Diagram

The Prisma Flow diagram is presented in **Fig. 1**. Searches identified a total of 18,542 articles for screening with an additional 9 articles identified via the reference lists from systematic reviews. After duplicates were removed a total of 8567 unique titles and abstracts were screened for inclusion. After title and abstract screening, 300 full-text articles were retrieved and screened for inclusion. A total of 252 full-text articles were excluded because they included the wrong age group (n = 100), measured only one season (n = 80), were gray literature (n = 43), could not be located (n = 9), were a review article (n = 8), were not published in English (n = 8), or did not include physical activity or sleep outcomes (n = 5). Thus, 47 articles were included in the narrative synthesis and meta-analysis.

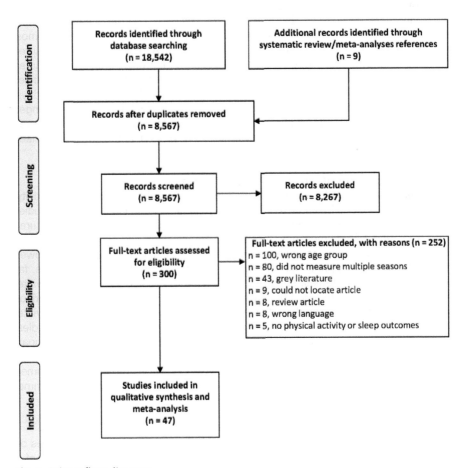

Fig. 1. Prisma flow diagram.

Narrative Synthesis

Study characteristics

Study characteristics are reported in **Table 1**. A total of 2 studies were conducted in Asia, 23 studies were conducted in Europe, 18 studies were conducted in North America, and 4 studies were conducted in Oceania. The 4 studies conducted in Oceania were the only studies conducted in the southern hemisphere. The latitudes of the studies conducted in the northern hemisphere ranged from 29 to 69°N, while the latitudes of the studies conducted in the southern hemisphere ranged from 31 to 37°S.

Sleep and activity monitoring methods and outcomes

A total of 40 studies measured physical activity only, 5 studies measured sleep only, and 2 studies measured sleep and physical activity. For physical activity, 6 studies measured sedentary behavior, 6 studies measured light physical activity, 7 studies measured MPA, 5 studies measured VPA, 10 studies measured MVPA, 12 studies measured steps, and 21 studies measured other physical activity. For sleep, 6 studies measured sleep duration, 2 studies measured sleep onset, 2 studies measured sleep offset, and 1 study measured sleep other (ie, parent reported if child sleeps more and is tired).

For physical activity, 36 studies included an objective measure while only 2 studies measuring sleep included an objective measure. The mean number of days of assessment of physical activity was 5.5 (SD = 2.5) and ranged from 1 to 14 days. The most common measurement duration was 7 days (16 studies). A total of 9 studies measured movement behaviors for 4 days, 4 studies measured for 5 days, 3 studies measured for 1 day, 3 studies measured for 2 days, 2 studies measured for 6 days, 2 studies measured for 9 days, and 1 study each measured for 1 day, 9 days, and 14 days. For sleep, the mean number of assessment days was 6.8 (SD = 5.1) and ranged from 1 to 14 days. A total of 2 studies measured sleep for 1 day, 2 studies measured sleep for 7 days, 2 studies measured sleep for 14 days, and 1 study measured sleep for 4 days.

Seasonal comparisons of physical activity and sleep

The seasons measured for each study are presented in **Table 1**. For physical activity, 18 studies measured 2 seasons, 12 studies measured 3 seasons, and 12 studies measured all 4 seasons. For sleep, 2 studies measured 2 seasons, 4 studies measured 3 seasons, and 1 study measured 4 seasons. Across sleep and physical activity, the most common behavior comparison was fall vs. spring with 31 studies, followed closely by winter vs. spring with 30 studies, then fall vs. winter with 25 studies, fall vs. summer with 21 studies, spring vs. summer with 22 studies, and finally winter vs. summer with 20 studies. For physical activity, the most common comparison was fall vs. spring with 27 studies, then winter vs. spring with 26 studies, fall vs. winter with 22 studies, spring vs. summer with 19 studies, fall vs. summer with 18 studies, and winter vs. summer with 17 studies. For sleep, the most common season comparison was fall vs. spring with 6 studies, followed by winter vs. spring with 5 studies. A total of 4 studies each compared children's sleep during fall vs. winter, fall vs. summer, and spring vs. summer. The least common sleep comparison was winter vs. summer with 3 studies.

Studies considering structure

When considering structure, a total of 17 of the 47 studies conducted measures on and presented outcomes separately for weekends and/or weekdays. A total of 8 studies measured summer during vacation from school while 1 study measured winter

Table 1
Table of included studies

Author, Year	Outcomes Measured	Obj Measure	Sample Size (n)	Female (n)	Country	Region	Lat	Study Design	Days Assessed (n)	Seasons Measured F	W	Sp	Su	Months Measured	Mean Age in Years (SD)	Vacation days Included During Fall[a]	Vacation days Included During Winter[a]	Vacation days Included During Spring[a]	Vacation days Included During Summer[a]	Week & Weekend Day[b]
Aadland, 2017[40]	LPA, MPA, MVPA, Sed, VPA	Yes	615	306	Norway	Europe	61.55°N	Cluster-randomized trial	7 d			●	●	Jan, Feb, Apr, May, Jun	10.9 (0.3)	Unclear	Unclear	Unclear	Unclear	Combined
Atkin, 2015[41]	MVPA, Sed	Yes	704	370	United Kingdom	Europe	52.18°N	Prospective observational	2 d	●	●	●	●	Jan, Feb, Mar, Apr, May, Jun, Jul, Aug, Sep, Oct, Nov, Dec	7.6 (0.3)	Unclear	Unclear	Unclear	Unclear	Separate
Bagordo, 2017[42]	PA other	No	250	123	Italy	Europe	43.73°N	Prospective observational	2 d	●			●	NR (winter, and late spring)	7.3 (0.9)	Unclear	Unclear	Unclear	Unclear	Combined
Beighle, 2008[43]	Steps	Yes	401	167	United States	North America	38.03°N	Prospective observational	4 d	●		●		Feb, May	9.1 (1.5)	No	No	No	No	Weekday only
Beighle, 2012[44]	Steps	Yes	105	65	United States	North America	38.03°N	Prospective observational	4 d	●	●			Feb, Oct	8.9 (0.7)	No	No	No	No	Weekday only
Brusseau, 2015[45]	PA other	Yes	289	168	United States	North America	40.76°N	Prospective observational	7 d	●			●	Apr, Oct	9.5 (0.7)	No		No		Separate
Carskadon, 1993[46]	Sleep other	No	1680	892	United States	North America	60.79°N to 28.53°N	Retrospective observational	1 d	●		●		Jan, Feb, Mar, Apr, May, Sep, Oct, Nov, Dec	10.5 (1.0)	No	No	No	No	Combined
Cooper, 2010[47]	PA other	Yes	1010	472	United Kingdom	Europe	51.45°N	Repeated cross-sectional	4 d	●	●	●	●	Jan, Feb, Mar, Apr, May, Jun, Jul, Aug, Sep, Oct, Nov, Dec	11.0 (0.4)	No	No	No	No	Weekday only
Cullen, 2017[48]	LPA, MVPA, Sed, Steps	Yes	342	342	United States	North America	29.76°N	Repeated cross-sectional	7 d	●	●	●	●	Jan, Feb, Mar, Apr, May, Jun, Jul, Aug, Sep, Oct, Nov, Dec	8–10 (–)	Unclear	Unclear	Unclear	Unclear	Combined

(continued on next page)

Table 1
(continued)

Author, Year	Outcomes Measured	Obj Measure Measured	Sample Size (n)	Female (n)	Country	Region	Lat	Study Design	Days Assessed (n)	Seasons Measured F	W	Sp	Su	Months Measured	Mean Age in Years (SD)	Vacation days Included During Fall[a]	Vacation days Included During Winter[a]	Vacation days Included During Spring[a]	Vacation days Included During Summer[a]	Week & Weekend Day[b]
Erwin, 1934[49]	Sleep duration	No	644	329	United States	North America	42.03°N	Repeated cross-sectional	7 d	●	●	●	●	Feb, May, July, Nov	8.5 (0.2)	Unclear	Unclear	Unclear	Unclear	Combined
Fu, 2017[50]	Steps	Yes	1232	624	United States	North America	39.54°N	Prospective observational	5 d	●			●	NR (beginning fall semester, end spring semester)	9.5 (1.8)	No	No	No	No	Weekday only
Harrison, 2017[51]	MVPA	Yes	591	302	United Kingdom	Europe	52.62°N	Prospective observational	2 d	●	●	●	●	Jan, Feb, Mar, Apr, May, Jun, Jul, Aug, Sep, Oct, Nov, Dec	7.3 (0.2)	Unclear	Unclear	Unclear	Unclear	Combined
Heelan, 2009[52]	PA other	Yes	123	73	United States	North America	41.27°N	Quasi-experimental	4 d	●	●	●		Feb, May, Aug	8.1 (1.7)	No	No	No	No	Weekday only
Hjorth, 2013[53]	Sleep duration, MVPA, Sed	Yes	730	354	Denmark	Europe	55.68°N	Prospective observational	4 d	●	●	●		Feb, Mar, Jun, Aug, Sep, Oct, Nov	10.0 (0.6)	No	No	No	No	Separate
Hopkins, 2011[54]	Steps, PA other	Yes	116	70	Australia	Oceania	31.98°S	Prospective observational	3 d	●				Jun, Nov	10.7 (0.3)	No			No	Combined
Kolle, 2009[55]	PA other	Yes	1291	598	Norway	Europe	60.47°N	Prospective observational	4 d	●	●	●		Jan, Feb, Mar, Apr, May, Jun, Sep, Oct, Nov	9.0 (–)	No	No	No	No	Combined
Kolle, 2008[56]	PA other	Yes	1127	525	Norway	Europe	60.47°N	Prospective observational	4 d	●	●	●		Jan, Feb, Mar, Apr, May, Jun, Sep, Oct, Nov	9.0 (–)	No	No	No	No	Combined
Kristensen, 2008[57]	PA other	Yes	793	437	Denmark	Europe	55.40°N	Repeated cross-sectional	5 d	●	●	●	●	Mar, Apr, May, Jun, Aug, Sep, Oct, Nov, Dec	9.6 (0.4)	Unclear	Unclear	Unclear	Unclear	Combined

Study	Outcome		N (total)	N	Country	Continent	Latitude	Design	Days	Measurements	Months	Value					Timing
Langlois, 2012[58]	PA other	No	1206	627	Canada	North America	45.50°N	Prospective observational	7 d	●●●	Jan, Feb, Mar, Apr, May, Jun, Sep, Oct, Dec	12.3 (0.6)	No	No	No	No	Combined
Larouche, 2019[59]	PA other	No	932	516	Canada	North America	46.57°N	Prospective observational	7 d	●●●	NR	10.6 (0.7)	No	No	No	No	Weekday only
Loucaides, 2004[60]	Steps	Yes	144	71	Cyprus	Europe	35.19°N	Prospective observational	4 d	●	Jan, Feb, May, Jun	12.0 (–)	No	No	No	No	Weekday only
Loucaides, 2018[61]	Steps	Yes	73	37	Cyprus	Europe	34.71°N	Prospective observational	6 d	●●	Jan, May	11.5 (0.5)	No	No	No	No	Separate
Mattocks 2007[62]	PA other	Yes	315	167	United Kingdom	Europe	51.45°N	Prospective observational	7 d	●●●●	Mar, Apr, May, Jun, Jul, Aug, Sep, Oct, Nov, Dec	11.7 (0.2)	Unclear	Unclear	Unclear	Unclear	Combined
McCorie, 2017[63]	PA other	Yes	774	427	Scotland	Europe	56.49°N	Repeated cross-sectional	8 d	●●●●	Mar, Jun, Sep, Dec	10–11 (–)	Unclear	Unclear	Unclear	Unclear	Combined
McCorie, 2020[64]	MVPA	Yes	774	427	Scotland	Europe	55.87°N	Repeated cross-sectional	1 d	●●●●	Mar, Jun, Sep, Dec	11.1 (0.3)	Unclear	Unclear	Unclear	Unclear	Combined
Nagy, 2019[65]	PA other	Yes	104	53	United Kingdom	Europe	53.81°N	Prospective observational	9 d	●●●●	NR (3 school terms and 2 holiday terms)	7.5 (0.5)	No	No	No	Yes	Combined
Nilsen, 2019[66]	PA other	Yes	704	332	Norway	Europe	61.55°N	Prospective observational	4 d	●	Jan, Feb, March, Apr, May, Jun, Sep, Oct, Nov, Dec	5–6 (–)	No	No	No	No	Combined
Nixon, 2008[67]	Sleep duration	Yes	591	262	New Zealand	Oceania	37.92°S	Repeated cross-sectional	1 d	●●●●	Jan, Feb, March, Apr, May, Jun, Jul, Aug, Sep, Oct, Nov, Dec	7.3 (0.2)	Unclear	Unclear	Unclear	Unclear	Combined
Oreskovic, 2012[68]	PA other	Yes	24	14	United States	North America	42.41°N	Repeated cross-sectional	7 d	●●●	Mar, Jul, Dec	11–12 (–)	No	No	No	Yes	Combined

(continued on next page)

Table 1
(continued)

Author, Year	Outcomes Measured	Obj Measure	Sample Size (n)	Female (n)	Country	Region	Lat	Study Design	Days Assessed (n)	Seasons Measured F	W	Sp	Su	Months Measured	Mean Age in Years (SD)	Vacation days Included During Fall[a]	Vacation days Included During Winter[a]	Vacation days Included During Spring[a]	Vacation days Included During Summer[a]	Week & Weekend Day[b]
Ostrin, 2018[69]	Sleep duration, PA other	Yes	60	24	Unites States	North America	29.76°N	Prospective observational	14 d	●	●	●	●	Jan, Feb, March, Apr, May, Jun, Jul, Aug, Sep, Oct, Nov, Dec	7.6 (1.8)	No		No	Yes	Combined
Pagels, 2016[70]	PA other	Yes	179	87	Sweden	Europe	59.33°N	Prospective observational	5 d	●		●		Mar, May, Sep	10.2 (0.4)	No		No		Weekday only
Pagels, 2020[71]	PA other	Yes	159	78	Sweden	Europe	56.4°N to 60.3°N	Prospective observational	7 d	●		●		Mar, May, Sep	10.1 (0.5)	No	No	No	No	Weekday only
Remmers, 2017[72]	LPA, MPA, Sed, VPA	Yes	326	170	Australia	Oceania	37.81°S	Prospective observational	7 d	●	●	●	●	Feb, Mar, May, Jun, Aug, Sep, Oct, Nov	11.4 (0.7)	No	No	No	No	Combined
Ridgers, 2015[73]	MPA, MVPA, VPA	Yes	326	164	Australia	Oceania	37.81°S	Prospective observational	9 d	●	●	●	●	Feb, Mar, May, Jun, Aug, Sep, Oct, Nov	10.2 (0.7)	No	No	No	No	Combined
Rowlands, 2006[11]	Steps	Yes	36	0	England	Europe	51.31°N	Prospective observational	7 d		●		●	Jan, Feb, Jun, Jul	8.8 (0.8)	No	Yes	No	Yes	Separate
Rowlands, 2009[74]	MPA, VPA	Yes	64	39	United Kingdom	Europe	50.74°N	Prospective observational	6 d		●		●	Jan, Feb, Jun, Jul	9.9 (0.3)	No	No	No	No	Separate
Sethre-Hofstad, 2012[75]	Sleep duration, Sleep offset, Sleep onset	No	79	-	Norway	Europe	69°N	Prospective observational	7 d		●	●		Jan, May	7.7 (1.5)	No	No	No	No	Separate
Stevens, 2003[76]	PA other	No	683	329	United States	North America	34.05–43.97°N	Quasi-experimental	1 d	●				NR	8–12 (–)	No	Unclear	No	Yes	Weekday only
Szymczak, 1993[77]	Sleep duration, Sleep offset, Sleep onset	No	64	33	Poland	Europe	53.01°N	Prospective observational	14 d	●	●	●	●	Jan, Feb, March, Apr, May, Jun, Jul, Aug, Sep, Oct, Nov, Dec	10–12 (–)	Unclear	Unclear	Unclear	Unclear	Combined

Study	Measures	Obj	n	n	Country	Continent	Lat	Design	Duration	Seasons measured	Age				Week/weekend
Tanaka, 2016[78]	LPA, MPA, MVPA, Sed, Steps	Yes	209	111	Japan	Asia	35.58°N	Prospective observational	7 d	●● May, Jul, Aug	9.0 (1.8)	No	No	Yes	Combined
Tanaka, 2018[79]	LPA, MPA, MVPA, Steps, PA	Yes	209	111	Japan	Asia	35.58°N	Prospective observational	7 d	●● May, Jul, Aug	9.0 (1.8)	No	No	Yes	Combined
Vadiveloo, 2009[80]	Steps	Yes	32	24	United States	North America	42.36°N	Prospective observational	7 d	●●● Jan, Feb, May, Jun, Oct, Nov	9.5 (–)	No	No	No	Combined
Volmut, 2020[81]	LPA, MPA, MVPA, VPA	Yes	93	45	Slovenia	Europe	51.22°N	Prospective observational	5 d	●● May, Jun, Aug, Sep	7.6 (1.1)	No	No	Yes	Combined
Wickel, 2010[82]	Steps	Yes	80	38	United States	North America	36.15°N	Prospective observational	7 d	●● Jan, May, Sep	9.8 (0.9)	No	No		Separate
Ylitalo, 2019[83]	PA other	Yes	174	43	United States	North America	31.20°N	Prospective observational	7 d	● Jun, Jul, Aug, Sep, Oct, Nov, Dec	8.3 (1.6)	No		Yes	Combined
Zelener, 2016[84]	PA other	Yes	139	72	United States	North America	33.68°N	Prospective observational	1 d	● Apr, May, Sep, Oct	11.1 (0.4)	No	No	Yes	Combined
Sera, 2017[85]	PA other	Yes	6497	3321	United Kingdom	North America	55.38°N	Repeated cross-sectional	7 d	●●●● Jan, Feb, March, Apr, May, Jun, Jul, Aug, Sep, Oct, Nov, Dec	7.5 (–)	Unclear	Unclear	Unclear	Separate

Abbreviations: "Obj" Objective "Lat" Latitude, "LPA" light physical activity, "MPA" moderate physical activity, "MVPA" Moderate-to-vigorous Physical Activity, "PA Other" Physical Activity Other, "F" fall, "W" winter, "Sp" Spring, "Su" Summer.

a Yes = measures occurred during vacation from school (ie, winter, summer, spring vacation), No = measures occurred while children were attending school, Unclear = study does not present enough information to determine if measures occurred during vacation from school.

b Weekday only = only measured children on weekdays, combined = measured data on week and weekend days but presented a combined estimated, separate = presented separated estimates by week and weekend days for each season measured.

during vacation from school. No studies measured fall or spring during vacation from school.

Study quality

The risk of bias ratings by the study on all individual indicators is presented in **Fig. 2**. Overall, the scores ranged from 3 to 9 and the mean score was 6.8 (SD = 1.4) while the median score was 7.0. Indicators that were frequently rated as not meeting or could not be determined were, "was the participation rate of eligible persons at least 50%," "were inclusion and exclusion criteria for being in the study prespecified and applied uniformly to all participants," "was a sample size justification provided," "was loss to follow-up after baseline 20% or less," and "were key potential

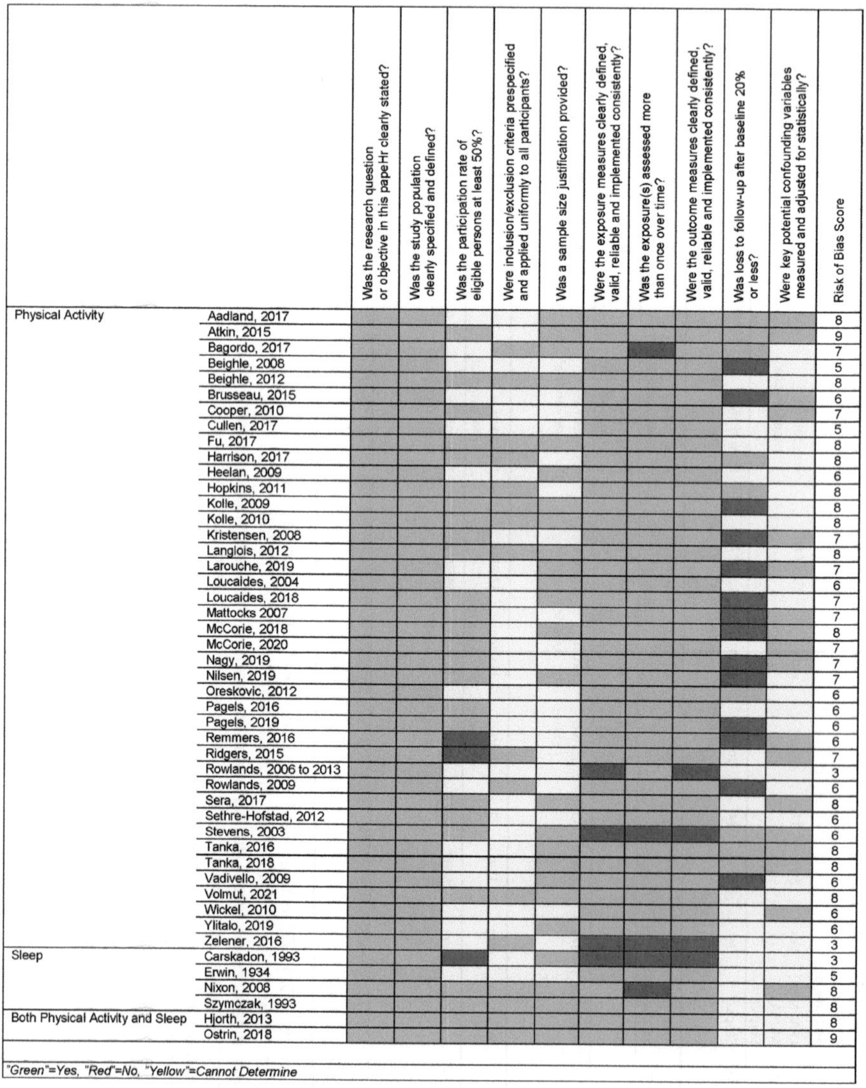

The columns are: Was the research question or objective in this paper/Hr clearly stated? | Was the study population clearly specified and defined? | Was the participation rate of eligible persons at least 50%? | Were inclusion/exclusion criteria prespecified and applied uniformly to all participants? | Was a sample size justification provided? | Were the exposure measures clearly defined, valid, reliable and implemented consistently? | Was the exposure(s) assessed more than once over time? | Were the outcome measures clearly defined, valid, reliable and implemented consistently? | Was loss to follow-up after baseline 20% or less? | Were key potential confounding variables measured and adjusted for statistically? | Risk of Bias Score

Category	Study	Risk of Bias Score
Physical Activity	Aadland, 2017	8
	Atkin, 2015	9
	Bagordo, 2017	7
	Beighle, 2008	5
	Beighle, 2012	8
	Brusseau, 2015	6
	Cooper, 2010	7
	Cullen, 2017	5
	Fu, 2017	8
	Harrison, 2017	8
	Heelan, 2009	6
	Hopkins, 2011	8
	Kolle, 2009	8
	Kolle, 2010	8
	Kristensen, 2008	7
	Langlois, 2012	8
	Larouche, 2019	7
	Loucaides, 2004	6
	Loucaides, 2018	7
	Mattocks 2007	7
	McCorie, 2018	8
	McCorie, 2020	7
	Nagy, 2019	7
	Nilsen, 2019	7
	Oreskovic, 2012	6
	Pagels, 2016	6
	Pagels, 2019	6
	Remmers, 2016	6
	Ridgers, 2015	7
	Rowlands, 2006 to 2013	3
	Rowlands, 2009	6
	Sera, 2017	8
	Sethre-Hofstad, 2012	6
	Stevens, 2003	6
	Tanka, 2016	8
	Tanka, 2018	8
	Vadivello, 2009	6
	Volmut, 2021	8
	Wickel, 2010	6
	Ylitalo, 2019	6
	Zelener, 2016	3
Sleep	Carskadon, 1993	3
	Erwin, 1934	5
	Nixon, 2008	8
	Szymczak, 1993	8
Both Physical Activity and Sleep	Hjorth, 2013	8
	Ostrin, 2018	9

"Green"=Yes, "Red"=No, "Yellow"=Cannot Determine

Fig. 2. Risk of bias scores for each study.

confounding variables measured and adjusted statistically for their impact on the relationship between exposure(s) and outcome(s)."

Meta-Analysis

Differences in activity levels and sleep by season

Table 2 presents the findings of the meta-regression analyses along with estimates of heterogeneity (ie, I^2 statistics). For PA, overall PA behaviors showed that spring was healthier than fall (SMD = -0.25, 95CI = $-0.26, -0.24$) with only MPA and VPA healthier in the fall. Overall spring was healthier than winter (SMD = -0.35, 95CI = -0.36, -0.34) with only MPA and VPA showing no difference between spring and winter. Spring was healthier than summer when considering overall PA behaviors (SMD = -0.03, 95CI = $-0.05, -0.01$), LPA, MPA, steps, and TPA. However, summer was healthier than spring when considering MVPA and there was no difference between spring and summer for VPA, sedentary time, or PA other.

Overall fall was healthier than winter (SMD = -0.17, 95CI = $-0.18, -0.16$) with MPA, sedentary, steps, TPA, and PA other being consistent with the overall finding. LPA, VPA, and MVPA showed no difference between fall and winter. Overall, summer was healthier than fall (SMD = 0.15, 95CI = 0.13, 0.18). However, findings on specific PA behaviors were mixed with MPA and VPA being healthier in the fall but MVPA, sedentary, TPA, and PA Other being healthier in the summer. Overall, summer was healthier than the winter (SMD = 0.12, 95CI = 0.10, 0.14). Again, findings for specific PA behaviors were mixed with MPA and VPA being healthier in the winter and MVPA, sedentary, steps, TPA, and PA Other being healthier in the summer.

For sleep, overall sleep was healthier in the fall compared with spring (SMD = 0.10, 95CI = 0.05, 0.15). Sleep was also healthier in the winter compared with spring (SMD = 0.32, 95CI = 0.27, 0.36). Both sleep duration and sleep offset followed this pattern when comparing spring to winter, but no difference was found between the 2 seasons for sleep onset. Overall summer was healthier than spring for sleep as well (SMD = 0.74, 95CI = 0.66, 0.83). When comparing fall to winter, fall to summer, and winter to summer, the only sleep behavior measured was sleep duration. These findings indicated that sleep duration was not different between fall and winter and was healthier in the summer compared with the fall (SMD = 1.56, 95CI = 1.43, 1.68) and in the summer compared with the winter (SMD = 0.72, 95CI = 0.61, 0.84).

Table 2
Meta-regression effects of season by physical activity and sleep outcome

	Spring vs. Fall				Spring vs. Winter				Spring vs. Summer				Fall vs. Winter				Fall vs. Summer				Winter vs. Summer			
	n	k	I^2	eff	95CI	k	n	I^2	eff	95CI	k	n	I^2	eff	95CI	k	n	I^2	eff	95CI	k	n	I^2	eff	95CI	k	n	I^2	eff	95CI

Physical Activity

Overall	24	96	98.0	**-0.25**	**(-0.26, -0.24)**	25	139	96.9	**-0.35**	**(-0.36, -0.34)**	16	64	92.0	**-0.03**	**(-0.05, -0.01)**	18	88	93.9	**-0.17**	**(-0.18, -0.16)**	12	57	95.5	**0.15**	**(0.13, 0.18)**	14	100	93.2	**0.12**	**(0.10, 0.14)**
LPA	2	2	66.6	**-0.15**	**(-0.26, -0.05)**	3	4	0.0	**-0.12**	**(-0.20, -0.04)**	4	5	76.4	**-0.29**	**(-0.38, -0.20)**	2	2	0.0	0.07	(-0.04, 0.18)	2	2	59.9	-0.04	(-0.14, 0.07)	3	13	0.0	-0.06	(-0.15, 0.02)
MPA	2	5	97.2	**0.37**	**(0.30, 0.34)**	3	7	95.0	-0.01	(-0.07, 0.05)	4	8	86.5	**-0.11**	**(-0.17, -0.05)**	2	5	92.6	**-0.11**	**(-0.18, -0.04)**	2	5	90.8	**-0.33**	**(-0.40, -0.26)**	3	20	8.9	**-0.17**	**(-0.23, -0.11)**
VPA	2	5	96.1	**0.32**	**(0.25, 0.39)**	3	7	97.5	-0.03	(-0.09, 0.03)	3	6	93.7	0.01	(-0.06, 0.07)	2	5	93.3	-0.01	(-0.08, 0.06)	2	5	44.9	**-0.28**	**(-0.35, -0.21)**	3	20	52.1	**-0.19**	**(-0.25, -0.13)**
MVPA	7	20	98.8	**-0.47**	**(-0.50, -0.44)**	9	32	98.0	**-0.39**	**(-0.42, -0.37)**	9	21	94.4	**0.08**	**(0.05, 0.12)**	6	18	98.1	-0.02	(-0.04, 0.01)	6	14	97.3	**0.33**	**(0.29, 0.37)**	6	15	97.3	**0.20**	**(0.16, 0.23)**
Sed	4	6	89.5	-0.10	(-0.15, -0.05)	5	8	95.2	**-0.17**	**(-0.21, -0.12)**	4	5	13.9	-0.05	(-0.12, 0.02)	4	6	49.3	**-0.15**	**(-0.20, -0.11)**	4	5	90.5	**0.23**	**(0.16, 0.30)**	3	3	95.8	**0.33**	**(0.25, 0.41)**
Steps	4	12	78.0	**-0.24**	**(-0.30, -0.19)**	4	12	60.4	**-0.34**	**(-0.43, -0.25)**	3	4	77.1	**-0.48**	**(-0.59, -0.37)**	4	19	77.3	**-0.18**	**(-0.25, -0.11)**	2	4	85.0	-0.02	(-0.14, 0.10)	3	7	97.5	**0.31**	**(0.20, 0.42)**
TPA	7	11	97.8	**-0.48**	**(-0.51, -0.44)**	7	18	97.8	**-0.72**	**(-0.76, -0.69)**	3	8	92.9	**-0.17**	**(-0.29, -0.04)**	6	10	81.1	**-0.29**	**(-0.33, -0.26)**	4	17	48.4	**0.25**	**(0.18, 0.32)**	3	11	89.7	**0.21**	**(0.09, 0.32)**
PA Other	7	35	97.7	**-0.21**	**(-0.23, -0.20)**	9	51	93.6	**-0.35**	**(-0.37, -0.33)**	4	7	54.0	-0.02	(-0.08, 0.04)	3	23	51.9	**-0.23**	**(-0.24, -0.21)**	2	5	95.2	**0.43**	**(0.37, 0.50)**	4	9	93.8	**0.42**	**(0.36, 0.48)**

Sleep

Overall	6	38	90.3	0.10	(0.05, 0.15)	5	52	90.5	**0.32**	**(0.27, 0.36)**	4	28	96.0	**0.74**	**(0.66, 0.83)**	3	26	62.9	0.00	(-0.05, 0.06)	3	19	91.3	**1.56**	**(1.43, 1.68)**	2	18	73.2	**0.72**	**(0.61, 0.84)**
Sleep Duration	6	32	91.8	**0.12**	**(0.07, 0.17)**	5	34	91.9	**0.40**	**(0.35, 0.45)**	4	22	94.4	**1.32**	**(1.21, 1.43)**	3	26	62.9	0.00	(-0.05, 0.06)	3	19	91.3	**1.56**	**(1.43, 1.68)**	2	18	73.2	**0.72**	**(0.61, 0.84)**
Sleep Onset	-	-	-	-	-	2	9	82.3	-0.07	(-0.18, 0.04)	-	-	-	-	-	-	-	-	-	-	-	-	-	-	-	-	-	-	-	-	-
Sleep Offset	-	-	-	-	-	2	9	69.1	**0.35**	**(0.24, 0.46)**	-	-	-	-	-	-	-	-	-	-	-	-	-	-	-	-	-	-	-	-	-

Abbreviations: "n" number of studies, "k" number of effects, "eff" effect, "LPA" Light Physical Activity, "MPA" Moderate Physical Activity, "VPA" Vigorous Physical Activity, "MVPA" Moderate-to-vigorous Physical Activity, "Sed" Sedentary, "PA Other" Physical Activity Other.
Bolded text indicates statistically significant value at p<0.05.

Favors Fall	Favors Winter	Favors Spring	Favors Summer		

Changes in the activity level and sleep by season when considering structure

Findings on weekdays and weekends are presented in **Table 3** and were similar in magnitude and direction except for overall physical activity in fall compared with winter. The only comparison that was substantively different was fall compared with winter. During weekdays fall was healthier than winter (SMD = −0.11, 95CI = −0.16, −0.05) while there was a nonstatistical SMD of 0.02 (95CI = −0.03, 0.07) in favor of the winter on weekend days. Given the lack of studies measuring during vacation from school in the fall, winter, and spring meta-analytic comparisons between summer and other seasons were the only comparisons possible. When examining these analyses **(Table 4)**, a pattern emerged whereby physical activity was less healthy (ie, direction of difference changes and/or magnitude of difference grew) during the months of summer when physical activity was measured while school was not in session. Specifically, overall physical activity during the summer was healthier than spring when physical activity was measured during the months of summer while school was in session (SMD = 0.03, 95CI = 0.00, 0.05). However, spring was healthier than the summer when physical activity was measured during the months of summer while school was not in session (SMD = −0.46, 95CI = −0.54, −0.39). This pattern was consistent for all physical activity outcomes when comparing spring to summer. Only one study compared winter to summer when school was not in session so meta-analyses were not completed. There were no studies comparing fall to summer that measured physical activity during the months of summer when school was not in session. For sleep, only one study measured sleep during the summer when school was not in session so meta-analyses were not completed. Findings indicated that when sleep was measured during the months of summer and school was in session, summer was healthier than spring (SMD = 0.74, 95CI = 0.65, 0.83).

DISCUSSION

This systematic review and meta-analysis sought to summarize the difference between children's movement behaviors by season. Overall, it seems that children engaged in the healthiest levels of sedentary behavior and physical activity in the spring and the healthiest levels of sleep in the summer, although this varied for specific physical activity and sleep behaviors. It seems that structure during a given season may play a large role in the variation in children's movement behaviors. Thus, the findings above may be confounded by structure. However, the evidence in this area is limited as very few studies measured children when they were not in school during

Table 3
Meta-regression effects of seasons on weekend and weekdays

		Spring vs. Fall			Spring vs. Winter				Fall vs. Winter				Winter vs. Summer			
		n	k	effect	95CI		k	n	effect	95CI		k	n	effect	95CI		k	n	effect	95CI
Physical Activity																
Overall	Weekday	2	7	-0.51	(-0.56, -0.46)	2	7	-0.57	(-0.62, -0.52)	2	7	-0.11	(-0.16, -0.05)	2	26	0.09	(-0.01, 0.18)
	Weekend	2	7	-0.39	(-0.44, -0.34)	2	7	-0.54	(-0.59, -0.49)	2	11	0.02	(-0.03, 0.07)	2	26	0.11	(0.01, 0.20)
Sleep																
Overall	Weekday	.	.	.	.	2	10	0.42	(0.34, 0.50)	.	.	.	.	.	.	.	.
	Weekend	.	.	.	.	2	9	0.34	(0.26, 0.42)	.	.	.	.	.	.	.	.
Duration	Weekday	.	.	.	.	2	4	0.54	(0.43, 0.64)	.	.	.	.	.	.	.	.
	Weekend	.	.	.	.	2	3	0.43	(0.32, 0.54)	.	.	.	.	.	.	.	.

Abbreviations: "n" number of studies, "k" number of effects, "SMD" Standardized Mean Difference, "LPA" Light Physical Activity, "MPA" Moderate Physical Activity, "VPA" Vigorous Physical Activity, "MVPA" Moderate-to-vigorous Physical Activity, "Sed" Sedentary, "PA Other" Physical Activity Other.
Bolded text indicates statistically significant value at p<0.05

Favors Fall		Favors Winter		Favors Spring		Favors Summer	

Table 4
Meta-regression effects of seasons compared to summer when considering structure

	Spring vs. Summer				Fall vs. Summer				Winter vs. Summer			
	n	k	effect	95CI	n	k	effect	95CI	n	k	effect	95CI
All PA Metrics												
Summer Structure	14	28	**0.03**	**(0.00,** | **0.05)**	14	46	**0.12**	**(0.10,** | **0.14)**	14	86	**0.07**	**(0.05,** | **0.09)**
No Summer Structure	2	15	**-0.46**	**(-0.54,** | **-0.39)**	-	-	-	-	-	-	-	-	-	-
Light PA												
Summer Structure	2	2	**-0.20**	**(-0.30,** | **-0.09)**	2	2	-0.04	(-0.14, | 0.07)	3	14	-0.06	(-0.15, | 0.02)
No Summer Structure	2	3	**-0.50**	**(-0.65,** | **-0.34)**	-	-	-	-	-	-	-	-	-	-
Moderate PA												
Summer Structure	2	5	-0.06	(-0.13, | 0.01)	2	5	**-0.33**	**(-0.40,** | **-0.26)**	3	21	**-0.17**	**(-0.23,** | **-0.11)**
No Summer Structure	2	3	**-0.38**	**(-0.53,** | **-0.22)**	-	-	-	-	-	-	-	-	-	-
Vigorous PA												
Summer Structure	2	5	0.04	(-0.02, | 0.11)	2	5	**-0.28**	**(-0.35,** | **-0.21)**	3	21	**-0.19**	**(-0.25,** | **-0.13)**
No Summer Structure	-	-	-	-	-	-	-	-	-	-	-	-	-	-
MVPA												
Summer Structure	7	12	**0.11**	**(0.07,** | **0.14)**	6	12	**0.33**	**(0.29,** | **0.37)**	6	12	**0.21**	**(0.17,** | **0.25)**
No Summer Structure	2	3	**-0.46**	**(-0.62,** | **-0.30)**	-	-	-	-	-	-	-	-	-	-
Sedentary												
Summer Structure	3	3	-0.03	(-0.11, | 0.04)	4	4	**0.25**	**(0.18,** | **0.33)**	3	3	**0.33**	**(0.25,** | **0.41)**
No Summer Structure	-	-	-	-	-	-	-	-	-	-	-	-	-	-
Steps												
Summer Structure	-	-	-		-	2	4	-0.02	(-0.14,	0.10)	3	5	**0.17**	**(0.05,**	**0.28)**
No Summer Structure	2	3	**-0.67**	**(-0.83,** | **-0.51)**	-	-	-	-	-	-	-	-	-	-
Total PA												
Summer Structure	-	-	-		-	4	15	**0.30**	**(0.22,**	**0.38)**	3	4	0.02	(-0.21,	0.25)
No Summer Structure	-	-	-	-	-	-	-	-	-	-	-	-	-	-
PA Other												
Summer Structure	-	-	-		-	-	-	-		-	4	6	**0.16**	**(0.05,** | **0.27)**
No Summer Structure	-	-	-	-	-	-	-	-	-	-	-	-	-	-
All Sleep Metrics												
Summer Structure	3	27	**0.74**	**(0.65,** | **0.83)**	2	18	**1.77**	**(1.64,** | **1.90)**	2	18	**0.72**	**(0.61,** | **0.84)**
No Summer Structure	-	-	-	-	-	-	-	-	-	-	-	-	-	-
Sleep Duration												
Summer Structure	-	-	-		-	2	18	**1.77**	**(1.64,**	**1.90)**	2	18	**0.72**	**(0.61,**	**0.84)**
No Summer Structure	-	-	-	-	-	-	-	-	-	-	-	-	-	-

Abbreviations: "n" number of studies, "k" number of effects, "SMD" Standardized Mean Difference, "Lat" Latitude, "PA Other" Physical Activity Other.
Bolded text indicates statistically significant value at p<0.05

Favors Fall		Favors Winter		Favors Spring		Favors Summer	

summer vacation and even fewer studies made comparisons on weekdays and weekends between seasons.

This systematic review and meta-analysis extend previous reviews of the literature on seasonal change in movement behaviors in several key ways. First, previous reviews have focused on physical activity exclusively, with no reviews examining the variation in children's sleep behaviors by season.[2–5] Second, previous systematic reviews have not used meta-analytic approaches to combine study estimates.[2–5] Rather studies have P-value counted to draw conclusions about the impact of season on children's movement behaviors. This is a limitation of previous studies because this approach is highly subjective, focuses on the statistical significance of findings rather than the magnitude of the effect, and there is no way to correct for study features such as study design and sample characteristics.[16,17] Finally, this systematic review accounted for structure when considering the difference in children's movement behaviors across seasons. Structure has been shown to impact children's physical activity and sleep behaviors[18,19] and is critical to consider when examining shifts in children's movement behaviors by season.

The current study found that children's physical activity was the healthiest during the spring. This is a refinement of previous literature as we used meta-analytic techniques to estimate the magnitude of differences between seasons (rather than nominal significance). This refinement may, therefore, explain the contrasting results between previous findings, indicating that summer was the healthiest season for chidlren's physical activity. Further, the current review focused exclusively on children's movement behaviors rather than including all age groups (ie, adults, adolescents, and so forth).

The findings of this study, and previous systematic reviews on seasonal shifts in children's movement behaviors, call into question the validity of the findings of studies that evaluate interventions when baseline measures are conducted in one season and outcome measures in a different season (ie, baseline in the fall and outcome in the spring). This approach is common in large-scale physical activity interventions,[20–22] and is especially concerning given the findings of the current study indicate that physical activity is the healthiest in the spring. Thus, the findings of past studies should be considered in the context of seasonal variability of children's movement behaviors.

This is the first systematic review to specifically delineate the relation of structure with seasonal changes in children's movement behaviors. A major finding of this review is that very few studies have accounted for structure when exploring seasonal shifts in children's movement behaviors. This is a major gap in the literature. Only one study conducted measures while children were in school and on vacation from school during 2 different seasons.[11] This study measured 36 children on weekdays and weekends during winter vacation from school and winter school term and then measured the same children during summer vacation from school and summer term. The study found that children were generally most active during the summer vacation days on both weekdays and weekends. However, winter weekdays were more active than summer weekend days and were similarly active to summer weekdays. While the findings of this study are preliminary (ie, only 36 children) they highlight the impact that the presence or absence of the school day (ie, structure) may have on children's activity levels. These findings are also contradictory to the findings of the meta-analyses in this review whereby a pattern of less healthy physical activity levels emerged in studies that conducted summer measures when school was not in session compared with studies that conducted summer measures when school was in session. For instance, studies that conducted summer measures when school *was in session* showed that MVPA was healthier during the summer (SMD = 0.11, 95CI = 0.07, 0.14) compared with spring. However, studies that conducted summer measures when school *was not in session* showed that MVPA was less healthy during the summer (SMD = −0.46, 95CI = −0.62, −0.30) compared with spring. Nonetheless, these findings suggest that structure plays a major role in the physical activity of children and may override any seasonal variations that occur due to factors associated with season (ie, weather, photoperiod). However, more work with larger more representative samples of children that compare activity levels across seasons during vacation and school days is needed. This work is especially important as the popularity of year-round schools has grown in the United States, with 3700 year-round schools[23] serving more than 2,000,000 students across 45 states.[24] Year-round schools operate on a 180-day schedule, similar to traditional schools. However, year-round schools incorporate shorter, frequent breaks throughout the calendar year rather than taking one prolonged 2–3-month break over summer. Thus, understanding the interaction of structure and seasonal changes in children's physical activity, sedentary behaviors, and sleep is critically important for this small but growing subgroup of children.

This systematic review also found that sleep duration is the healthiest in the summer. This is surprising given that the photoperiod is the longest in the summer compared with the other months of the year, and thus, suggests that children should be sleeping for shorter durations compared with other seasons that have shorter photoperiods. This is consistent with studies that have examined the impact of structure on children's sleep duration.[19,25] These studies show that children's sleep duration is longer when children are not in school, which typically occurs during the months of summer. In the current review, when considering structure for sleep, the data are sparse (ie, only 3 studies measured sleep outcomes during the months of summer while children were in school and 1 study measured sleep outcomes during the months of summer while children were not in school). Findings were mixed with all sleep metrics showing the minimal difference between seasonal changes in summer versus spring (SMD = 0.74 vs SMD = 0.80). However, sleep duration was considerably healthier during the summer compared with the spring (SMD = 1.37, 95CI = 1.25, 1.48) in the one study that conducted summer measures while children were in school. The SMD fell to 0.80 (95CI = 0.43,1.17) in the one study that compared spring and summer and conducted summer measures while children were not in school. Again, this pattern is consistent with past studies that show that children sleep less on school days compared with nonschool days.[19,25] This suggests that structure plays a major role in the sleep behaviors of children and may override any seasonal variations that occur due to photoperiod length. However, the evidence is limited and more studies that explore the impact of season and structure on children's sleep are needed.

This study has several strengths. The review presents a comprehensive synthesis of the literature exploring seasonal fluctuations in children's movement behaviors. The review focused on both sleep, sedentary behaviors, and physical activity to provide a comprehensive evaluation of the literature in this area. Further, minimal exclusion criteria were used to ensure that all pertinent studies were included. A meta-analysis was also performed to estimate the relationship of season with children's movement behaviors. Additionally, one must consider the current review in light of its limitations. Large heterogeneity was observed in study effects. This may have been due to the minimal inclusion/exclusion criteria, variability in participant inclusion criteria, heterogeneity in study protocols, and the widespread use of self-report measures.[26,27] Perhaps most notably, few studies considered the potential of structure to confound findings related to seasonal fluctuations in movement behaviors. Studies were either unclear when measures were conducted during the summer or conducted summer measures when children were on vacation from school. This is more a limitation of the current state of the literature than the current review. Future studies should be more transparent with reporting when measures are conducted, and future studies should consider structure when exploring seasonal changes in movement behaviors. Nonetheless, preliminary findings on the unique effects of structure versus season on children's movement behaviors highlight the need for future studies that explicitly measure and/or manipulate children's exposure to structure.

IMPLICATIONS FOR CLINICAL PRACTICE

The findings of this systematic review and meta-analysis have implications important implications for pediatric care. First, it is clear that children's behaviors vary seasonally. Thus, the timing of recommendations for increasing children's physical activity and reducing sedentary behaviors should coincide with these fluctuations (ie, recommendations for increasing physical activity and reducing sedentary behaviors before the summer months). Further linking children with structured activities when school is not in session could be critical for managing physical activity, sedentary behavior, and sleep and in-turn risk for overweight or obesity. The timing of clinic-based screenings for physical activity, sedentary behavior, and sleep at well-child visits is also crucial as screening occurs across seasons or during school vs. vacation may not be reliable or valid. Ideally, children's movement behaviors should be measured in multiple seasons. However, this is likely not feasible, and a suitable alternative is for screenings to be completed in the same season annually.

IMPLICATIONS FOR INTERVENTION DESIGN

These findings are also crucial for the design and evaluation of interventions targeting children's movement behaviors. Similar to clinic-based screenings studies evaluating interventions to impact children's movement behaviors should measure children's behaviors in multiple seasons before and following the intervention. At the very least, measurements should be completed in the same season before and following the intervention. Second, interventions targeting children's physical activity during the winter and fall (when children are in school) and during the summer (when children are not in school) may have a greater impact on children's physical activity behaviors given that children are already the most active during the spring. Third, there were surprisingly few studies that examined seasonal changes in children sleep behaviors, and even fewer studies examining metrics outside of sleep duration. Understanding seasonal shifts children's sleep timing and consistency (unique from duration) have both been shown to be related to overweight and obesity risk independent of sleep duration[28–31] may be salient targets for interventions to improve children's sleep. Finally, the data from this systematic review indicated that seasonal shifts in children's physical activity behavior, specifically those during the summer, are dependent on the presence of the school day. This can likely be explained by the structured days' hypothesis that posits that the presence of the school day positively impacts children's health behaviors.[18] These findings combined with recent studies showing that children's physical activity levels decreased during school closures,[32–36] and subsequent studies showing children's BMI gain increased during the COVID-19 pandemic,[37–39] bolster the argument that school positively impacts children's movement behaviors, and these positive behaviors mitigate unhealthy BMI gain. This information can inform when interventions targeting children's movement behaviors should be delivered and may provide novel intervention strategies (ie, providing access to structured programs during unstructured times).

CLINICS CARE POINTS

- Timing of recommendations for increasing children's physical activity and reducing sedentary behaviors should coincide with children's fluctuations in physical activity, sedentary behaviors, and sleep (ie, recommendations for increasing physical activity and reducing sedentary behaviors before the summer months).

- Linking children to structured activities when school is not in session could be critical for managing physical activity, sedentary behavior, and sleep and in-turn risk for overweight or obesity.

- Screenings for physical activity, sedentary behavior, and sleep at well-child visits should be completed in the same season annually.

POTENTIAL CONFLICTS OF INTEREST

The authors have nothing to disclose.

FUNDING

Research reported in this publication was supported by the National Institute of General Medical Sciences of the National Institutes of Health under Award Number 1P20GM130420 The content is solely the responsibility of the authors and does not necessarily represent the official views of the National Institutes of Health.

ACKNOWLEDGMENTS

None

SUPPLEMENTARY DATA

Supplementary data related to this article can be found online at https://doi.org/10.1016/j.pcl.2022.04.005.

REFERENCES

1. Rollo S, Antsygina O, Tremblay MS. The whole day matters: understanding 24-hour movement guideline adherence and relationships with health indicators across the lifespan. J Sport Health Sci 2020.
2. Tucker P, Gilliland J. The effect of season and weather on physical activity: a systematic review. Public Health 2007;121(12):909–22.
3. Turrisi TB, Bittel KM, West AB, et al. Seasons, weather, and device-measured movement behaviors: a scoping review from 2006 to 2020. Int J Behav Nutr Phys Act 2021;18(1):1–26.
4. Rich C, Griffiths LJ, Dezateux C. Seasonal variation in accelerometer-determined sedentary behaviour and physical activity in children: a review. Int J Behav Nutr Phys Act 2012;9:49.
5. Carson V, Spence JC. Seasonal variation in physical activity among children and adolescents: a review. Pediatr Exerc Sci 2010;22(1):81–92.
6. Brazendale K, Beets M, Pate RR, et al. Understanding differences between summer vs. school obesogenic behaviors of children: the structured days hypothesis. Int J Behav Nutr Phy 2017;14(1):100.
7. Moher D, Liberati A, Tetzlaff J, et al. Preferred reporting items for systematic reviews and meta-analyses: the PRISMA statement. PloS Med 2009;6(7):e1000097.
8. Page MJ, Moher D, Bossuyt PM, et al. PRISMA 2020 explanation and elaboration: updated guidance and exemplars for reporting systematic reviews. BMJ 2021;372.
9. Higgins JP, Thomas J, Chandler J, et al. Cochrane handbook for systematic reviews of interventions. John Wiley & Sons; 2019.
10. National Institutes of Health. Study quality assessment tools. Available at. https://www.nhlbi.nih.gov/health-topics/study-quality-assessment-tools. Accessed May 17, 2021.
11. Rowlands AV, Hughes DR. Variability of physical activity patterns by type of day and season in 8-10-year-old boys. Res Q Exerc Sport 2006;77(3):391–5.
12. Hedberg E. ROBUMETA: Stata module to perform robust variance estimation in meta-regression with dependent effect size estimates 2014.

13. Tufanaru C, Munn Z, Stephenson M, et al. Fixed or random effects meta-analysis? Common methodological issues in systematic reviews of effectiveness. Int J Evid Based Healthc 2015;13(3):196–207.

14. Ryan R. Cochrane consumers and communication group: meta-analysis. Cochrane Consumers and Communication Review Group; 2016.

15. Benjamini Y, Hochberg Y. Controlling the false discovery rate: a practical and powerful approach to multiple testing. J R Stat Soc Ser B (Methodological) 1995;57(1):289–300.

16. Cheung MW-L, Vijayakumar R. A guide to conducting a meta-analysis. Neuropsychol Rev 2016;26(2):121–8.

17. Cooper H, Hedges LV, Valentine JC. The handbook of research synthesis and meta-analysis. Russell Sage Foundation; 2019.

18. Brazendale K, Beets MW, Weaver RG, et al. Understanding differences between summer vs. school obesogenic behaviors of children: the structured days hypothesis. Int J Behav Nutr Phys Act 2017;14(1):100.

19. Weaver R, Armstrong B, Hunt E, et al. The impact of summer vacation on children's obesogenic behaviors and body mass index: a natural experiment. Int J Behav Nutr Phys Act 2020;153.

20. Folta SC, Kuder JF, Goldberg JP, et al. Changes in diet and physical activity resulting from the Shape Up Somerville community intervention. BMC Pediatr 2013; 13:157.

21. Sallis JF, McKenzie TL, Alcaraz JE, et al. The effects of a 2-year physical education program (SPARK) on physical activity and fitness in elementary school students. sports, play and active recreation for kids. Am J Public Health 1997; 87(8):1328–34.

22. Luepker RV, Perry CL, McKinlay SM, et al. Outcomes of a field trial to improve children's dietary patterns and physical activity: the child and adolescent trial for cardiovascular health (CATCH). JAMA 1996;275(10):768–76.

23. Skinner RR. Year-round schools: in brief 2014. Available at. https://fas.org/sgp/crs/misc/R43588.pdf. Accessed February 25, 2017.

24. McGlynn A. Districts That School Year-Round. 2002. Available at. http://www.aasa.org/SchoolAdministratorArticle.aspx?id=10416. Accessed February 25, 2017.

25. Weaver RG, Beets MW, Perry M, et al. Changes in children's sleep and physical activity during a 1-week versus a 3-week break from school: A natural experiment. Sleep 2019;42(1):zsy205.

26. O'Brien KT, Vanderloo LM, Bruijns BA, et al. Physical activity and sedentary time among preschoolers in centre-based childcare: a systematic review. Int J Behav Nutr Phys Act 2018;15(1):117.

27. Hnatiuk JA, Salmon J, Hinkley T, et al. A review of preschool children's physical activity and sedentary time using objective measures. Am J Prev Med 2014; 47(4):487–97.

28. Golley RK, Maher CA, Matricciani L, et al. Sleep duration or bedtime? Exploring the association between sleep timing behaviour, diet and BMI in children and adolescents. Int J Obes (Lond) 2013;37(4):546–51.

29. Jarrin DC, McGrath JJ, Drake CL. Beyond sleep duration: distinct sleep dimensions are associated with obesity in children and adolescents. Int J Obes 2013;37(4):552.

30. Arora T, Taheri S. Associations among late chronotype, body mass index and dietary behaviors in young adolescents. Int J Obes 2015;39(1):39.

31. Olds TS, Maher CA, Matricciani L. Sleep duration or bedtime? Exploring the relationship between sleep habits and weight status and activity patterns. Sleep 2011;34(10):1299–307.

32. Moore SA, Faulkner G, Rhodes RE, et al. Impact of the COVID-19 virus outbreak on movement and play behaviours of Canadian children and youth: a national survey. Int J Behav Nutr Phys Act 2020;17(1):1–11.

33. Burkart S, Parker H, Weaver RG, et al. Impact of the COVID-19 pandemic on elementary schoolers' physical activity, sleep, screen time and diet: A quasi-experimental interrupted time series study. Pediatr Obes 2021;e12846.

34. Bates LC, Zieff G, Stanford K, et al. COVID-19 Impact on behaviors across the 24-hour day in children and adolescents: physical activity, sedentary behavior, and sleep. Children 2020;7(9):138.

35. Hemphill NM, Kuan MTY, Harris KC. Reduced physical activity during COVID-19 pandemic in children with congenital heart disease. Can J Cardiol 2020;36(7): 1130–4.

36. Okely A, Kariippanon K, Guan H, et al. Global effect of COVID-19 pandemic on physical activity, sedentary behaviour and sleep among 3-to 5-year-old children: a longitudinal study of 14 countries. 2020.

37. Weaver RG, Hunt ET, Armstrong B, et al. COVID-19 leads to accelerated increases in children's BMI z-score gain: An interrupted time-series study. Am J Prev Med 2021;61(4):e161–9.

38. Browne NT, Snethen JA, Greenberg CS, et al. When pandemics collide: The impact of COVID-19 on childhood obesity. J Pediatr Nurs 2020;56(90).

39. Woolford SJ, Sidell M, Li X, et al. Changes in body mass index among children and adolescents during the COVID-19 pandemic. JAMA 2021;326(14):1434–6.

40. Aadland E, Andersen LB, Skrede T, et al. Reproducibility of objectively measured physical activity and sedentary time over two seasons in children; comparing a day-by-day and a week-by-week approach. PLoS One 2017;12(12):e0189304.

41. Atkin AJ, Sharp SJ, Harrison F, et al. Seasonal variation in children's physical activity and sedentary time. Med Sci Sports Exerc 2016;48(3):449–56.

42. Bagordo F, De Donno A, Grassi T, et al. Lifestyles and socio-cultural factors among children aged 6-8 years from five Italian towns: the MAPEC_LIFE study cohort. BMC Public Health 2017;17(1):233.

43. Beighle A, Alderman B, Morgan CF, et al. Seasonality in children's pedometer-measured physical activity levels. Res Q Exerc Sport 2008;79(2):256–60.

44. Beighle A, Erwin H, Morgan CF, et al. Children's in-school and out-of-school physical activity during two seasons. Res Q Exerc Sport 2012;83(1):103–7.

45. Brusseau TA. The intricacies of children's physical activity. J Hum Kinet 2015;47: 269–75.

46. Carskadon MC, Acebo C. Parental reports of seasonal mood and behavior changes in children. J Am Acad Child Adolesc Psychiatry 1993;32(2):264–9.

47. Cooper AR, Page AS, Wheeler BW, et al. Patterns of GPS measured time outdoors after school and objective physical activity in English children: the PEACH project. Int J Behav Nutr Phys Act 2010;7:31.

48. Cullen KW, Liu Y, Thompson D. Diet and physical activity in african-american girls: seasonal differences. Am J Health Behav 2017;41(2):171–8.

49. Erwin D. An analytical study of children's sleep. Pedagogical Seminary J Genet Psychol 1934;45(1):199–226.

50. Fu Y, Brusseau TA, Hannon JC, et al. Effect of a 12-week summer break on school day physical activity and health-related fitness in low-income children from CSPAP schools. J Environ Public Health 2017;2017.

51. Harrison F, Atkin AJ, van Sluijs EMF, et al. Seasonality in swimming and cycling: exploring a limitation of accelerometer based studies. Prev Med Rep 2017; 7:16–9.

52. Heelan KA, Abbey BM, Donnelly JE, et al. Evaluation of a walking school bus for promoting physical activity in youth. J Phys Act Health 2009;6(5):560–7.

53. Hjorth MF, Chaput JP, Michaelsen K, et al. Seasonal variation in objectively measured physical activity, sedentary time, cardio-respiratory fitness and sleep duration among 8-11 year-old Danish children: a repeated-measures study. BMC Public Health 2013;13:808.

54. Hopkins N, Stratton G, Ridgers ND, et al. Lack of relationship between sedentary behaviour and vascular function in children. Eur J Appl Physiol 2012;112(2): 617–22.

55. Kolle E, Steene-Johannessen J, Andersen LB, et al. Seasonal variation in objectively assessed physical activity among children and adolescents in Norway: a cross-sectional study. Int J Behav Nutr Phys Act 2009;6:36.

56. Kolle E, Steene-Johannessen J, Andersen LB, et al. Objectively assessed physical activity and aerobic fitness in a population-based sample of Norwegian 9- and 15-year-olds. Scand J Med Sci Sports 2010;20(1):e41–7.

57. Kristensen PL, Korsholm L, Møller NC, et al. Sources of variation in habitual physical activity of children and adolescents: the European youth heart study. Scand J Med Sci Sports 2008;18(3):298–308.

58. Langlois KA, Birkett N, Garner R, et al. Trajectories of physical activity in Montreal adolescents from age 12 to 17 years. J Phys Act Health 2012;9(8):1146–54.

59. Larouche R, Gunnell K, Bélanger M. Seasonal variations and changes in school travel mode from childhood to late adolescence: a prospective study in New Brunswick, Canada. J Transport Health 2019;12:371–8.

60. Loucaides CA, Chedzoy SM, Bennett N. Differences in physical activity levels between urban and rural school children in Cyprus. Health Educ Res 2004;19(2): 138–47.

61. Loucaides CA. Seasonal differences in segmented-day physical activity and sedentary behaviour in primary school children. Early Child Development Care 2018;188(3):410–20.

62. Mattocks C, Leary S, Ness A, et al. Intraindividual variation of objectively measured physical activity in children. Med Sci Sports Exerc 2007;39(4):622–9.

63. McCrorie P, Mitchell R, Ellaway A. Comparison of two methods to assess physical activity prevalence in children: an observational study using a nationally representative sample of Scottish children aged 10-11 years. BMJ open 2018;8(1): e018369.

64. McCrorie P, Mitchell R, Macdonald L, et al. The relationship between living in urban and rural areas of Scotland and children's physical activity and sedentary levels: a country-wide cross-sectional analysis. BMC Public Health 2020; 20(1):304.

65. Nagy LC, Horne M, Faisal M, et al. Ethnic differences in sedentary behaviour in 6-8-year-old children during school terms and school holidays: a mixed methods study. BMC Public Health 2019;19(1):152.

66. Nilsen AKO, Anderssen SA, Ylvisaaker E, et al. Physical activity among Norwegian preschoolers varies by sex, age, and season. Scand J Med Sci Sports 2019;29(6):862–73.

67. Nixon GM, Thompson JM, Han DY, et al. Short sleep duration in middle childhood: risk factors and consequences. Sleep 2008;31(1):71–8.

68. Oreskovic NM, Blossom J, Field AE, et al. Combining global positioning system and accelerometer data to determine the locations of physical activity in children. Geospat Health 2012;6(2):263–72.
69. Ostrin LA, Sajjadi A, Benoit JS. Objectively measured light exposure during school and summer in children. Optom Vis Sci 2018;95(4):332–42.
70. Pagels P, Raustorp A, Guban P, et al. Compulsory school in- and outdoors-implications for school children's physical activity and health during one academic year. Int J Environ Res Public Health 2016;13(7).
71. Pagels P, Wester U, Mårtensson F, et al. Pupils' use of school outdoor play settings across seasons and its relation to sun exposure and physical activity. Photodermatol Photoimmunol Photomed 2020;36(5):365–72.
72. Remmers T, Thijs C, Timperio A, et al. Daily weather and children's physical activity patterns. Med Sci Sports Exerc 2017;49(5):922–9.
73. Ridgers ND, Salmon J, Timperio A. Too hot to move? objectively assessed seasonal changes in Australian children's physical activity. Int J Behav Nutr Phys Act 2015;12:77.
74. Rowlands AV, Pilgrim EL, Eston RG. Seasonal changes in children's physical activity: an examination of group changes, intra-individual variability and consistency in activity pattern across season. Ann Hum Biol 2009;36(4):363–78.
75. Sethre-Hofstad L, Dahl TI. Arctic larks and owls: children's sleeping patterns north of the arctic circle. Individual Differences Res 2012;10(1):1–18.
76. Stevens J, Story M, Ring K, et al. The impact of the pathways intervention on psychosocial variables related to diet and physical activity in American Indian schoolchildren. Prev Med 2003;37(6 Pt 2):S70–9.
77. Szymczak J, Jasińska M, Pawlak E, et al. Annual and weekly changes in the sleep-wake rhythm of school children. Sleep 1993;16(5):433–5.
78. Tanaka C, Reilly JJ, Tanaka M, et al. Seasonal changes in objectively measured sedentary behavior and physical activity in Japanese primary school children. BMC Public Health 2016;16(1):969.
79. Tanaka C, Reilly JJ, Tanaka M, et al. Changes in weight, sedentary behaviour and physical activity during the school year and summer vacation. Int J Environ Res Public Health 2018;15(5).
80. Vadiveloo M, Zhu L, Quatromoni PA. Diet and physical activity patterns of school-aged children. J Am Diet Assoc 2009;109(1):145–51.
81. Volmut T, Pišot R, Planinšec J, et al. Physical activity drops during summer holidays for 6-to 9-year-old children. Front Public Health 2020;8.
82. Wickel EE, Welk GJ. Applying generalizability theory to estimate habitual activity levels. Med Sci Sports Exerc 2010;42(8):1528–34.
83. Ylitalo KR, Bridges CN, Gutierrez M, et al. Sibship, physical activity, and sedentary behavior: a longitudinal, observational study among Mexican-heritage sibling dyads. BMC Public Health 2019;19(1):1–9.
84. Zelener J, Schneider M. Adolescents and self-reported physical activity: An evaluation of the modified Godin Leisure-time exercise questionnaire. Int J Exerc Sci 2016;9(5):587.
85. Sera F, Griffiths LJ, Dezateux C, et al. Using functional data analysis to understand daily activity levels and patterns in primary school-aged children: cross-sectional analysis of a UK-wide study. PLoS One 2017;12(11):e0187677.

Effectively Supporting Youth with Chronic Illness in Schools
External Partnerships and Training Recommendations

Brian P. Daly, PhD[a],*, Shannon Litke, BA[a], Jenna Kiely, BA[b],
Paul C. Jones, PhD[c], Katelyn Wargel, MA MPA[d],
Paul Flaspohler, PhD[d], Kathryn Mancini, PhD[e]

KEYWORDS

- Childhood chronic health conditions • School • Academic functioning
- School performance • Behavioral health • Socioemotional health • School personnel
- Interdisciplinary collaboration

KEY POINTS

- One-fifth of school-aged children and adolescents have a childhood chronic health condition (CHC) that may impact their academic functioning, school performance, and behavioral and socioemotional health.
- School personnel such as teachers and counselors frequently report inadequate training to support the educational and psychosocial needs of these youth.
- Training in supporting youth with CHCs should be provided to graduate and preprofessionals who plan to work in school settings.
- Interdisciplinary collaboration and models of coordinated care have shown promise in effectively supporting youth with CHCs in school settings.

[a] Department of Psychological and Brain Sciences, Drexel University, 3141 Chestnut Street, Philadelphia, PA 19104, USA; [b] PolicyLab and the Center for Pediatric Clinical Effectiveness, Children's Hospital of Philadelphia (CHOP), 734 Schuylkill Avenue, Philadelphia, PA 19146, USA; [c] Temple University, 1301 Cecil B. Moore Avenue, Philadelphia, PA 19122, USA; [d] Miami University, 90 N Patterson Avenue, Oxford, OH 45056, USA; [e] MetroHealth Medical Center, Case Western Reserve University School of Medicine, 2500 MetroHealth Drive, Cleveland OH 44019, USA
* Corresponding author.
E-mail address: bpd36@drexel.edu

Pediatr Clin N Am 69 (2022) 695–707
https://doi.org/10.1016/j.pcl.2022.04.013
0031-3955/22/© 2022 Elsevier Inc. All rights reserved.

DISEASE-LEVEL, SCHOOL-LEVEL, SYSTEMS-LEVEL ISSUES

Childhood chronic health conditions (CHCs) generally refer to a disease state that has symptoms with a protracted course and involves one or more organ systems (eg, brain, heart, lung, blood) and may impair health status, psychological functioning, or academic performance.[1] Conditions are defined as chronic when they persist for more than 3 months within 1 year, affect the child's typical functioning and normal activities, and require ongoing care from one or more health care providers.[1] Across Western countries, prevalence data indicate that approximately 15% to 20% of school-aged children and adolescents suffer from a health-related disorder,[2] with incidence rates of CHCs in children continuing to increase. A significant subset of these children will experience negative consequences related to their health condition, including impaired academic functioning and school performance.[3] In addition, children with CHCs are at greater risk for emotional, social, and behavioral problems relative to their healthy peers.[4] These issues represent significant challenges for school-aged children, yet many school-based personnel including teachers and counselors report inadequate training to work with youth with CHCs.[5] Developing competencies to effectively support students with CHCs represent a key challenge for teachers and behavioral health professionals working in school settings.[6]

Although CHCs may be managed medically, they are rarely able to be completely cured and often persist for extended periods and sometimes for life.[1] Some children and adolescents with a CHC and their families experience high levels of psychosocial and educational stress and consequently require substantial amounts of time, energy, and personal resources to cope with the stressors and demands associated with their illness. For these reasons, effectively supporting youth with CHCs in schools is a multifaceted challenge that requires the attention and expertise of individuals from a variety of disciplines including psychology, psychiatry, pediatrics, medical specialists, counseling, and social work.

Disease-level issues: Some examples of CHCs seen in school settings include (but are not limited to) asthma, birth defects, type 1 and type 2 insulin-dependent diabetes mellitus, congenital heart disease, juvenile rheumatoid arthritis, cerebral palsy, muscular dystrophy, sickle cell disease, hemophilia, cystic fibrosis, cancer, head injuries, epilepsy, spina bifida, and human immunodeficiency virus. Stressors and challenges associated with CHCs can be conceptualized as disease related or treatment related. Children and adolescents with CHCs often must negotiate multiple disease-related stressors that include initial diagnosis and related testing, complex regimen adherence, pain, disrupted sleep, symptom flare-ups, and missing school due to medical complications.[7] These stressors are frequently associated with psychosocial and educational challenges such as changes in cognition, mood (depression, anxiety), behavior, social relationships, confidence, self-esteem, and academic performance.

Treatment-related stressors: In some CHCs such as cancer, diabetes, and sickle cell disease, neurocognitive changes occur because of the disease and/or the treatment and associated toxicities. These changes contribute to decreased educational performance and reduced quality of life among children and adolescents with CHCs.[8] Although affected cognitive domains vary by disease pathophysiology and treatment type, higher-order cognitive skills such as attention, executive function, learning, visuospatial skills, and memory are most frequently negatively impacted. For example, children with cancer may be treated with surgical intervention, cranial radiation therapy, and/or central nervous system (CNS) chemotherapy. Each of these treatments modalities may confer adverse long-term CNS-related outcomes including deficits in attention, learning, and memory.[8] Youth with sickle cell disease may experience neurologic complications including strokes and silent infarcts that result in cognitive impairments most prominently affecting attention, concentration, memory, and executive function.[9] The neurocognitive deficits found across disease types negatively impact learning and academic achievement, thereby compromising educational attainment and future vocational opportunities[10] and highlighting the need for effective coordination among school and medical professionals.

District- and school-level issues: School districts are legally responsible for setting policies, guidance, and protocols that are responsive to the needs of students. "Other health impairment" is one of the 14 categories of disability listed in special education law, the Individuals with Disabilities Education Act (IDEA). Under IDEA, a child who has an "other health impairment" is very likely to be eligible for special services to help the child address his or her educational, developmental, and functional needs resulting from the disability. For youth with CHCs, these special services and associated policies need to attend to medical concerns, challenges with adherence, and learning issues. These policies also must be sensitive to confidentiality of health care information and provide a roadmap for appropriate training of school personnel on the impacts of CHCs at school and school-related activities. Districts are similarly responsible for monitoring whether schools are following the various policies, guidance, and protocols intended to provide a safe and supportive educational environment for students with CHCs.

At the school-building level, students with CHCs first need to be identified and health care records requested and reviewed to determine which supports and accommodations are responsive to student needs. A 504 Plan, Individualized Education Plan (IEP), or other school plan such as the Individualized Healthcare Plan should be developed in collaboration with the family, student (if appropriate), school health staff (eg, nurse), primary and specialty health care providers, learning support coordinator, counselor, and teacher. The resulting accommodations and recommendations should specify the roles and responsibilities of specific school staff in making sure the health, behavioral health, and educational needs are being met for the identified student. Schools share the responsibility of ongoing communication with the family and health care providers as well as frequent monitoring and updating (as needed) of the plan.

Systems-level issues: There are many systems involved in effectively supporting youth with CHCs, including the family, school, primary and specialty health care providers, and community organizations that require coordinated strategies across multiple levels and sectors to best support youth. Evolving approaches include extending the scope of health care systems and services to new settings such as school-based health clinics and developing partnerships between schools and community health organizations to address health behaviors. Although each of these models has unique advantages and disadvantages, there is a constant need for frequent and meaningful communication between the family, health care provider, and the school that focus on student-centered problem solving.[10]

TRAINING NEEDS AND PROFESSIONAL DEVELOPMENT

Considering the prevalence and impact of CHCs among school-aged youth, it is important for appropriate professional development and training measures to be established for students in the allied health professions (eg, medicine, social work, psychology), as well as in-service training for school personnel (eg, teachers, administrators). Such training frameworks should be continually adapted to address barriers to implementing practice guidelines for integrated care.

Training Needs of Medical and Mental Health Professionals

It is important that graduate-level training programs in medicine, psychology, and social work include an explicit instructional framework in their curricula to prepare future care providers for the level of interdisciplinary collaboration required to support youth with CHCs in schools. One style of training is interprofessional education, whereby students from 2 or more allied health professions are grouped together as part of a shared learning process with the goal of promoting collaborative practice.[11] Specifically, interprofessional education focuses on instilling core competencies involving teamwork, knowledge of roles, communication, and values and ethics.[12,13] Although there is some evidence that interprofessional education in medical school is associated with improved clinical decision making and quality of care, firm conclusions on the overall effectiveness of this training approach are limited by the paucity of large-scale research studies and variability across curricula for different programs.[14]

The American Psychological Association's Society of Pediatric Psychology (Division 54) commissioned a Task Force to define core competencies that operationalize the training needs of graduate-level students in pediatric psychology.[15] Of the 10 "cross-cutting knowledge competencies" outlined,[15] 2 domains relate to the goal of interprofessional collaboration in supporting youth with CHCs in school settings. Specifically, these guidelines propose that pediatric psychologists should be trained to understand "the roles of other disciplines in health service delivery systems," as well as "how other systems (eg, school, health care, state and federal policies) affect pediatric health and illness and a child's adaptation to that illness."[15] Recommendations from the Division 54 Task Force further specified operational definitions for these applied competencies in terms of behavioral markers of graduate students' readiness for practicum, internship, and entry to practice. For example, according to these competency standards, pediatric psychologists' readiness to enter professional practice is measured in part by their ability to "independently design and implement systems interventions in the context of clinical work."[15] These competencies are intended to serve as recommendations to aid academic institutions in the development of appropriate graduate-level training experiences.

Although there are clearly established frameworks for providing comprehensive, interdisciplinary graduate education to providers serving youth with CHCs, barriers to implementation still exist in professional practice, suggesting a need for more targeted training. In a recent systematic review, Nooteboom and colleagues[16] identified barriers associated with implementing an integrated care model for youth including unclear or competing professional roles, lack of provider self-efficacy when addressing higher-severity problems, unfamiliarity with other professionals' care systems and protocols, and fragmentation stemming from differences in culture and procedures between school professionals (eg, teachers) and professionals from other health care settings.[16] Although these findings suggest that further training and support are required to bridge these gaps in professional competency, research has shown that there is no single model or universal approach to successfully implementing integrated care.[17] As such, training in integrative care models requires flexible adaptation based on local and individual needs.[18] Nooteboom and colleagues[16] recommend giving professionals an active, collaborative role in the development of their graduate-level training methods as a way to increase applicability of content and promote effective practice.

In tandem with explicit training on interprofessional collaboration and integrated care, it is imperative that allied health professionals, including psychologists, receive graduate-level training on how the biological correlates and medical management of specific pediatric CHCs affect practice parameters across domains.[15] An understanding of the medical profiles of CHCs is a crucial component of selecting and delivering appropriate psychosocial interventions and supports that fit the diverse needs of these youth.[19]

In-Service Training for School Personnel

Even though most school personnel report having contact with at least 1 student with a CHC in their school, findings from a survey of more than 1000 teachers revealed that only 8% reported receiving adequate training to assist youth with CHCs in the classroom, with the majority (52.3%) reporting receiving no training at all.[20] Research on teacher training programs has shown that providing educators with specific content designed to increase their awareness of CHCs had a significant impact on their level of knowledge in this area.[21] Therefore, curricula structured to address this gap should be developed and disseminated as a standardized component of professional development for teachers and other school personnel.

According to a comprehensive review of curricula for various teacher preparation programs in the United States, required preprofessional coursework for teachers largely failed to include content directly related to CHCs.[5] Instead, this topic was grouped under the category of "other health impairment" in the context of training in special education criteria.[5] In the absence of a basic level of training to enhance awareness of CHCs, teachers are left with misconceptions about which students fall within this definitional category. These misconceptions may result in teachers struggling to identify and implement appropriate supports.[5] For example, teachers may perceive students with CHCs to be at higher risk for experiencing medical complications in the classroom, thus increasing risk of liability and shifting teacher attention to mitigating this risk. However, students with CHCs also are at a higher risk of developing psychosocial and learning difficulties.[22] Without proper training to prepare and support teachers to recognize and correct this response pattern, there is a risk of unintentionally exacerbating the level of isolation and learning difficulties experienced by some of these students. As discussed by Irwin and colleagues,[5] it is likely that current programmatic training deficits are a symptom of larger-scale structural issues (eg, inconsistent terminology and lack of definitional criteria for CHCs, varied prevalence estimates). As such, it is recommended that policies are developed to address systems-level barriers to support youth with CHCs. For example, Valentijn and colleagues[23] emphasize the important role of "normative integration," whereby mutual shared goals and missions are clearly defined and disseminated by leaders across sectors to promote coherence and consistency between disciplines.

EVIDENCE-BASED PREVENTION AND INTERVENTION STRATEGIES FOR YOUTH WITH CHRONIC HEALTH CONDITIONS

A social model approach to prevention and intervention strategies for youth with CHCs places an emphasis on the systemic issues and barriers, rather than on the family and child.[24] This approach requires frequent communication between the family, school staff, and medical professionals regarding the child's health status, needs, and challenges. Consent for external medical providers to speak to school administrators directly eases the burden on caregivers, allowing administrators to then relay communications to the teachers.[24]

Physical Well-being

The physical well-being and safety of students with CHCs should be considered the main priority.[25] School staff that interact with the child, including teachers, the principal, medical personnel, and aides, should learn more about the child's CHC. These personnel should be aware of signs of symptom flare-ups and needed accommodations.[26] Students also may experience residual concerns due to the CHC, such as physical or mental impairments, fatigue, pain, or even behavior problems. Thus, accommodations should be addressed holistically, rather than focusing solely on direct symptoms.[24,25] Staff should also be trained on emergency protocols such as how to help a child with epilepsy having a seizure.

There is some evidence to suggest that providing age-appropriate, strengths-based education to children about their CHC can empower them while also decreasing overall symptoms.[26,27] For example, in a sample of Latino and African American students, participants randomized to receive an 8-week educational and coaching intervention on asthma management had fewer days of symptom exacerbation, and even fewer emergency room visits compared with students who did not receive the intervention.[26] Halterman and colleagues[27] found similar effects with a sample of 3- to 10-year-olds. These findings highlight the importance of including the child in the management of their own physical well-being, even during early childhood.

Academic Well-being

For children unable to regularly attend school, offering remote opportunities to engage in school can help maintain a sense of routine and identity as a student, rather than solely as a patient.[10,28] Developing individualized academic plans with input from caregivers and the IEP team at school can be especially helpful for children with inconsistent attendance or those on a homebound placement. These plans ideally allow for flexibility as needed while also providing structure to foster educational advancement. Teachers may assume that children with CHCs who are frequently absent would want less work, but teachers' reluctance to assign homework may further marginalize these students from their classmates and negatively impact their education attainment.[10] Homebound services for children with CHCs should be provided in a manner that supports appropriate access and reasonable rigor during times of chronic conditions. Wilkie and Jones[24] recommend that teachers, students, and their families directly discuss keeping up with schoolwork, and then set short-term and realistic goals. Importantly, when a determination is made for a homebound placement, the IEP team should set a reasonable time for review of the placement.

Socioemotional Well-being

Schools are key settings for fostering socioemotional well-being among children with CHCs. Negative peer relationships, or low social support, can exacerbate symptoms of chronic illness.[29] For example, negative peer interactions can impact glucose levels, which is dangerous for children with diabetes.[25] Therefore, it is recommended that children be encouraged to have open, teacher-facilitated discussions about their CHC with their classmates, which can increase the child's sense of empowerment and decrease stigma.[25,29]

INTERDISCIPLINARY COLLABORATION AND MODELS OF COORDINATED CARE FOR MEDICALLY COMPROMISED YOUTH

There is broad consensus that partnership between schools and health care providers is beneficial to meeting the physical and mental health needs of children in schools.[30,31] Although not without its challenges, there are many school-based opportunities for intervention and monitoring of children with CHCs to improve physical, psychosocial, and academic outcomes.[32] Strong interdisciplinary teams for the coordination of care between home, school, and community partners are critical.[33]

The biomedical model of disease and the myopic focus on symptoms of disease is widely viewed as inadequate for the treatment and management of chronic health problems.[34] The biopsychosocial model of illness developed out of the need for a broader conceptualization of disease. From a social-ecological perspective,[35,36] child development occurs not in isolation, but in the context of multiple interacting systems around the child including family, health care systems, and educational systems proximal to the child and cultural and social norms distally.[37]

Given the interaction between family, health care, and educational systems in the care of a child with a CHC, a coordinated approach to intervention is crucial. The need for interdisciplinary collaboration is emphasized by health profession advocacy groups. The American Academy of Pediatrics,[38] for example, acknowledges the complexity of the educational system and encourages its members to seek out additional systems-level advocacy and training regarding the accessibility of education for children with disabilities and CHCs. Despite such policy statements and the perceived benefit of collaboration, the actual frequency and quality of collaboration pediatricians engage in with school professionals remain subject to various barriers, including the lack of training in collaboration.[39]

Interdisciplinary Collaborative Models

Drotar and colleagues[40] emphasize the role of pediatric psychologists in care coordination for individuals with CHCs across health care settings and schools, summarizing several models of consultation. At a fundamental level, each individual professional fulfills their respective role, but there is otherwise limited interaction between professionals. Other models involve more ongoing consultation for the management of a problem between professionals, either indirectly or through interdisciplinary collaboration with shared responsibility and decision making among professionals.

The need for coordination across systems is highlighted across various models of interdisciplinary collaboration. Walsh and colleagues[41] proposed a developmental approach as a theoretic framework from which to guide interprofessional collaboration. The eco-triadic model of consultation highlights the interaction between families, health care professionals, and school professionals by way of an educational consultant.[42] The biopsychoeducational model of consultation was developed to guide school psychologists toward acting as liaison between systems, using an ecological framework.[43] Sheridan and colleagues[44] developed conjoint behavioral consultation to promote positive family-school relationships. Conjoint behavioral consultation has demonstrated good empirical support in consultation across home and school settings.[45,46] This model has been extended to interdisciplinary collaboration with health care professionals, as well.[47] Conjoint behavioral consultation services were implemented for physician-referred children, with consultants (trained school psychology graduate students) providing liaison services to families, medical providers, and school professionals. Results were encouraging, suggesting efficacy of conjoint behavioral consultation services for promoting interdisciplinary care and goal attainment among children with CHCs and their families.

Practical considerations related to interdisciplinary collaboration and care coordination remain. The difficulties related to lack of training in effective models of collaboration have been expounded earlier. In addition, cost is often cited as a barrier to implementation, as consultation services are rarely reimbursed by insurance companies.[31,40] To overcome such barriers, pediatricians may need to seek out additional training opportunities in collaborating with schools, engage in systems-level change related to school and medical-home collaboration, and use other health and human services personnel (eg, nursing staff, physician extenders, medical home behavioral health staff) to improve communication and care coordination.[38,39] Medical homes must find other efficient means of coordinating care with school systems. For example, creating draft letters for use by physicians and parents to communicate medical findings to schools can improve communication.[48] The use of goal attainment scales can be an efficient means to communicate progress between stakeholders.[49] From a professional standpoint, roles should be clarified among professionals and collaborators should be viewed as equal partners.[41]

School-Based Health Centers

School-based health centers (SBHCs) have become an increasingly more common model of providing health care services to students with and without CHCs. Within the context of an SBHC, interdisciplinary collaboration between medical and educational professionals is improved for children with CHCs.[32] Colocating health care services in schools can support interdisciplinary collaboration and coordinated care, increase access to health care services, improve health care utilization, and improve economic costs of health care.[50] Among low-income youth, SBHCs have demonstrated a positive relationship with increased school connectedness.[51] Through school connectedness, SBHCs have been indirectly associated with improved academic performance, but not attendance.[52] Despite such opportunities for collaboration, establishing ties between family, school, and health providers remains a challenge even within SBHCs.[53]

Even with the recognition that interdisciplinary collaboration is critical for the coordination of care, the aforementioned models rarely offer specific criteria or guidance for conducting such consultation between systems. In addition, there are several barriers to interdisciplinary collaboration, including time, financial reimbursement, and training.[31,40] Power and Blom-Hoffman[32] highlight both opportunities and challenges associated with implementing health interventions in school settings. Schools offer the benefit of a naturalistic environment to develop, implement, and monitor progress under the supervision of a multidisciplinary team. Professionals in schools, however, often lack appropriate training and expertise related to needs of medically compromised students, whereas health care professionals lack training and expertise in educational systems.[32,54] Despite differences in areas of expertise, there is agreement for the need for increased consultation across systems. Pediatricians recognize the importance of collaboration with schools and engage in infrequent consultation with schools, primarily with teachers.[39] Similarly, school psychologists reported infrequent collaboration with pediatricians.[30]

A developmentally focused, social-ecological model is useful to understand the effects of CHCs on children. Using a systems framework, families, health professionals, and school personnel can engage in interdisciplinary collaboration to identify early signs of risk and promote health and well-being by evaluation and intervention within and between systems.[55] Despite several models of interdisciplinary collaboration for the purposes of coordinated care for medically compromised youth, there remains a significant gap in translating models into practice. Methodological issues exist in evaluating the effectiveness of such models, including that of SBHCs.[56,57]

SUMMARY AND FUTURE DIRECTIONS

One-fifth of school-aged children and adolescents have a CHC that may impact their academic functioning, school performance, and behavioral and socioemotional health.[2] School personnel such as teachers and counselors frequently report inadequate training to support the educational and psychosocial needs of these youth. Therefore, trainings and policies should be developed at the school- and district-level that are responsive to the continuing education needs of these professionals. At the pipeline level, training in supporting youth with CHCs should be provided to graduate and preprofessionals who plan to work in school settings. Educational activities for current professionals and trainees should emphasize interdisciplinary collaboration and models of coordinated care to best support youth with CHCs in school settings. Future research should seek to better understand how to best translate these models into practice while also evaluating the effectiveness of such models.

CLINICS CARE POINTS

- Multidisciplinary team members such as a specialist in education, psychologist, a speech and language pathologist, a physical therapist, an occupational therapist, and/or a physician who work with youth with CHCs should evaluate them for psychosocial and educational challenges as well as neurocognitive deficits, including changes in cognition, mood (depression, anxiety), behavior, social relationships, confidence, self-esteem, and academic performance.

- Children with CHCs should be comprehensively evaluated by school IEP teams to see if they qualify for "other health impairment", 1 of the 14 categories of disability listed in special education law, the IDEA.

- Under IDEA, a child who has an "other health impairment" may be eligible for special services to help the child address his or her educational, developmental, and functional needs resulting from the disability.

- At the point of clinical concern, parents, physicians, or other health service providers should refer children for a team evaluation and subsequent provision of services.

- To qualify for "other health impairment", a student must display evidence of the following criteria:
  ○ Limited strength as indicated by an inability to perform typical tasks at school
  ○ Limited vitality as indicated by an inability to sustain effort or to endure throughout an activity
  ○ Limited alertness as indicated by an inability to manage and maintain attention, to organize or attend, and to prioritize environmental stimuli, including heightened alertness to environmental stimuli that results in limited alertness with respect to the educational environment

- Trainees and professionals working with youth with CHCs should participate in interprofessional education programs that focus on instilling core competencies involving teamwork, knowledge of roles, communication, and values and ethics.

- Barriers associated with implementing an integrated care model for youth include[16]:
  ○ unclear or competing professional roles
  ○ lack of provider self-efficacy when addressing higher severity problems
  ○ unfamiliarity with other professionals' care systems and protocols
  ○ fragmentation stemming from differences in culture and procedures between school professionals (eg, teachers) and professionals from other health care settings

- Professionals should have an active, collaborative role in the development of training methods to increase applicability of content and promote effective practice at the local level

- Care coordination for individuals with CHCs across health care settings and schools should involve interdisciplinary collaboration with shared responsibility and decision making among professionals

- SBHCs represent a promising model of providing health care services to students with and without CHCs
- Barriers to interdisciplinary collaboration include time, financial reimbursement, and training[31,40]

DISCLOSURE STATEMENT

The authors report no commercial or financial conflicts of interest or additional funding sources.

REFERENCES

1. Wallander JL, Thompson RJ, Alriksson-Smith A. Psychosocial adjustment of children with chronic physical conditions. In: Roberts MC, editor. Handbook of pediatric psychology. 3rd edition. New York: Guildford; 2003. p. 141–58.
2. Center for Disease Control and Prevention. Summary of health statistics for U.S. children. Atlanta, Georgia: National Health Interview Survey; 2008.
3. Taras H, Potts-Datema W. Chronic health conditions and student performance at school. J Sch Health 2005;75(7):255–66.
4. Martinez YJ, Ercikan K. Chronic illnesses in Canadian children: what is the effect of illness on academic achievement, and anxiety and emotional disorders? Child Care Health Dev 2009;35(3):391–401.
5. Irwin MK, Elam M, Merianos A, et al. Training and preparedness to meet the needs of students with a chronic health condition in the school setting. Phys Disabilities Edu Relat Serv 2018;37(2):34–59.
6. Kaffenberger CJ. School reentry for students with a chronic illness: a role for professional school counselors. Prof Sch Couns 2006;9(3). https://doi.org/10.1177/2156759x0500900312.
7. Hains AA, Davies WH, Behrens D, et al. Cognitive behavioral interventions for adolescents with cystic fibrosis. J Pediatr Psychol 1997;22(5):669–87.
8. Compas BE, Jaser SS, Reeslund K, et al. Neurocognitive deficits in children with chronic health conditions. Am Psychol 2017;72(4):326–38.
9. Nicholls E, Hildenbrand AK, Aggarwal R, et al. The use of stimulant medication to treat neurocognitive deficits in patients with pediatric cancer, traumatic brain injury, and sickle cell disease: a review. Postgrad Med 2012;124(5):78–90.
10. Walcott CM, Harrison SE. Academic issues related to chronic health conditions in schools. In: Dempsey AG, editor. Pediatric health conditions in schools: guide for working with children, families, and educators. Oxford, United Kingdom: Oxford University Press; 2019.
11. Hammick M, Freeth D, Koppel I, et al. A best evidence systematic review of interprofessional education: BEME Guide no. 9. Med Teach 2007;29(8):735–51.
12. Interprofessional Education Collaborative Expert Panel. Core competencies for interprofessional collaborative practice: report of an expert panel. Washington, DC: Interprofessional Education Collaborative; 2011.
13. Thistlethwaite JE, Forman D, Matthews LR, et al. Competencies and Frameworks in Interprofessional Education. Acad Med 2014;89(6):869–75.
14. Vuurberg G, Vos JAM, Christoph LH, et al. The effectiveness of interprofessional classroom-based education in medical curricula: a systematic review. J Interprofessional Edu Pract 2019;15:157–67.

15. Palermo TM, Janicke DM, McQuaid EL, et al. Recommendations for training in pediatric psychology: defining core competencies across training levels. J Pediatr Psychol 2014;39(9):965–84.

16. Nooteboom LA, Mulder EA, Kuiper CHZ, et al. Towards Integrated Youth Care: A Systematic Review of Facilitators and Barriers for Professionals. Adm Policy Ment Health 2020;48(1). https://doi.org/10.1007/s10488-020-01049-8.

17. Curry N, Ham C. Clinical and service integration. *The route to improve outcomes*. London: The Kings Fund; 2010.

18. Dobbie M, Mellor D. Chronic illness and its impact: considerations for psychologists. Psychol Health Med 2008;13(5):583–90.

19. Selekman J. Students with chronic conditions: experiences and challenges of regular education teachers. J Sch Nurs 2016;33(4):307–15.

20. Brown MB, Bolen LM, Brinkman TM, et al. A collaborative strategy with medical providers to improve training for teachers of children with cancer. J Educ Psychol Consultation 2011;21(2):149–65.

21. Olson AL, Seidler AB, Goodman D, et al. School professionals' perceptions about the impact of chronic illness in the classroom. Arch Pediatr Adolesc Med 2004; 158(1):53–8.

22. Jackson M. The special educational needs of adolescents living with chronic illness: a literature review. Int J Inclusive Edu 2013;17(6):543–54.

23. Valentijn PP, Schepman SM, Opheij W, et al. Understanding integrated care: a comprehensive conceptual framework based on the integrative functions of primary care. Int J Integrated Care 2013;13:e010.

24. Wilkie K, Jones A. School ties: keeping students with chronic illness connected to their school learning communities. In: International federation for information processing (IFIP) conference. Laxenburg, Austria: International Federation for Information Processing; 2010. p. 1–13.

25. Guthrie DW, Bartsocas C, Jarosz-Chabot P, et al. Psychosocial issues for children and adolescents with diabetes: overview and recommendations. Diabetes Spectr 2003;16(1):7–12.

26. Bruzzese J-M, Sheares BJ, Vincent EJ, et al. Effects of a school-based intervention for urban adolescents with asthma. Am J Respir Crit Care Med 2011;183(8): 998–1006.

27. Halterman JS, Szilagyi PG, Fisher SG, et al. Randomized Controlled Trial to Improve Care for Urban Children With Asthma. Arch Pediatr Adolesc Med 2011;165(3). https://doi.org/10.1001/archpediatrics.2011.1.

28. Shaw L, Moore D, Nunns M, et al. Experiences of interventions aiming to improve the mental health and well-being of children and young people with a long-term physical condition: A systematic review and meta-ethnography. Child Care Health Dev 2019;45(6):832–49.

29. Saxby N, Beggs S, Battersby M, et al. What are the components of effective chronic condition self-management education interventions for children with asthma, cystic fibrosis, and diabetes? A systematic review. Patient Educ Couns 2019;102(4):607–22.

30. Bradley-Klug KL, Jeffries-DeLoatche KL, Walsh AStJ, et al. School psychologists' perceptions of primary care partnerships: implications for building the collaborative bridge. Adv Sch Ment Health Promotion 2013;6(1):51–67.

31. Shaw SR, Kelly DP, Joost JC, et al. School-linked and school-based health services: a renewed call for collaboration between school psychologists and medical professionals. Psychol Sch 1995;32(3):190–201.

32. Power TJ, Blom-Hoffman J. The school as a venue for managing and preventing health problems: Opportunities and challenges. In: Brown RT, editor. Handbook of pediatric psychology in school settings. Mahwah, New Jersey: Lawrence Erlbaum Associates, Inc; 2004. p. 37–48.

33. Shaw SR, McCabe PC. Hospital-to-school transition for children with chronic illness: Meeting the new challenges of an evolving health care system. Psychol Schools 2007;45(1):74–87.

34. Engel GL. The Need for a New Medical Model: A Challenge for Biomedicine. Holist Med 1989;4(1):37–53.

35. Bronfenbrenner U. Toward an experimental ecology of human development. Am Psychol 1977;32(7):513–31.

36. Kazak AE. Families of chronically ill children: a systems and social-ecological model of adaptation and challenge. J Consult Clin Psychol 1989;57(1):25–30.

37. Kazak AE, Alderfer MA, Reader SK. Families and other systems in pediatric psychology. In: Roberts MC, Steele RG, Alderfer MA, et al, editors. Handbook of pediatric psychology. 5th ed. New York, NY: Guilford Press; 2017.

38. Provision of educationally related services for children and adolescents with chronic diseases and disabling conditions. PEDIATRICS 2007;119(6):1218–23.

39. Bradley-Klug KL, Sundman AN, Nadeau J, et al. Communication and collaboration with schools: pediatricians' perspectives. J Appl Sch Psychol 2010;26(4): 263–81.

40. Drotar DD, Palermo TM, Barry C. Collaborating with schools: models and methods in pediatric psychology and pediatrics. In: Brown RT, editor. Handbook of pediatric psychology in school settings. Mahwah, New Jersey: Lawrence Erlbaum Associates, Inc; 2004. p. 21–36.

41. Walsh ME, Brabeck MM, Howard KA. Interprofessional collaboration in children's services: toward a theoretical framework. Children's Serv 1999;2(4):183–208.

42. Shields JD, Heron TE, Rubenstein CL, et al. The eco-triadic model of educational consultation for students with cancer. Edu Treat Child 1995;18(2):184–200. Available at: https://www.jstor.org/stable/pdf/42899401.pdf?refreqid=excelsior%3A72a6261b7e48b2ae7f726ecdb9f2bc4e. Accessed December 20, 2021.

43. Grier BC, Bradley-Klug KL. Collaborative consultation to support children with pediatric health issues: a review of the biopsychoeducational model. J Educ Psychol Consultation 2011;21(2):88–105.

44. Sheridan SM, Kratochwill TR, Burt JD. Conjoint behavioral consultation: promoting family-school connections and interventions. In: Conjoint behavioral consultation: promoting family-school connections and interventions. New York, NY: Springer Science+Bisomess Media, LLC.; 2010.

45. Sheridan SM, Eagle JW, Cowan RJ, et al. The effects of conjoint behavioral consultation results of a 4-year investigation. J Sch Psychol 2001;39(5):361–85.

46. Sheridan SM, Clarke BL, Knoche LL, et al. The effects of conjoint behavioral consultation in early childhood settings. Early Edu Dev 2006;17(4):593–617.

47. Sheridan SM, Warnes ED, Woods KE, et al. An exploratory evaluation of conjoint behavioral consultation to promote collaboration among family, school, and pediatric systems: a role for pediatric school psychologists. J Educ Psychol Consultation 2009;19(2):106–29.

48. Lewis JM, McCallister J, Browning S. ADHD parent–pediatrician letters to the school: a family-centered medical home tool to improve collaboration, grades, and behavior. Glob Pediatr Health 2015;2. https://doi.org/10.1177/2333794X15574284.

49. DuPaul GJ, Power TJ. Improving school outcomes for students with ADHD: Using the right strategies in the context of the right relationships. J Atten Disord 2008; 11:519–21.
50. Dunfee MN. School-based health centers in the United States: roots, reality, and potential. J Sch Health 2020;90(8). https://doi.org/10.1111/josh.12914.
51. Bersamin M, Coulter RWS, Gaarde J, et al. School-based health centers and school connectedness. J Sch Health 2018;89(1):11–9.
52. Strolin-Goltzman J, Sisselman A, Melekis K, et al. Understanding the relationship between school-based health center use, school connection, and academic performance. Health Soc Work 2014;39(2):83–91.
53. Meyers AB, Swerdlik ME. School-based health centers: opportunities and challenges for school psychologists. Psychol Schools 2003;40(3):253–64.
54. Sulkowski ML, Jordan C, Nguyen ML. Current practices and future directions in psychopharmacological training and collaboration in school psychology. Can J Sch Psychol 2009;24(3):237–44.
55. Power T. Collaborative practices for managing children's chronic health needs. In: Chronic health-related disorders in children: collaborative medical and psychoeducational interventions. Washington, DC: American Psychological Association; 2006.
56. Arenson M, Hudson PJ, Lee N, et al. The evidence on school-based health centers: a review. Glob Pediatr Health 2019;6. https://doi.org/10.1177/2333794x19828745.
57. Bersamin M, Garbers S, Gold MA, et al. Measuring success: evaluation designs and approaches to assessing the impact of school-based health centers. J Adolesc Health 2016;58(1):3–10.

Integrating Behavioral Health in Primary Care

Lessons from Interdisciplinary Collaboration in School Mental Health

Kathryn Mancini, PhD[a], Katelyn Wargel, MA, MPA[b],
Brian P. Daly, PhD[c], Shannon Litke, BA[c], Jenna Kiely, BA[d],
Paul Flaspohler, PhD[b],*

KEYWORDS

- Integrated primary care • Interdisciplinary team • Team capacity • Prevention
- Behavioral health promotion • Population-based care

KEY POINTS

- Integrated pediatric primary care (PPC) offers cost-efficient strategies to improve access to behavioral health care in primary care settings and has shown to be related to positive patient and provider outcomes.
- Barriers exist to widespread implementation of integrated PPC, generally related to lack of capacity to carry out integrated practice.
- The field of school mental health (SMH) has a wide body of research that provides some evidence for effective strategies to address behavioral health in school settings; 2 of these strategies may be relevant for IPC settings; (1) use of layered, interdisciplinary strategic and implementation teams and (2) a focus on using data to create population-based health promotion and intervention plans.

Concerns continue to grow around pediatric behavioral and mental health[1] (described together as behavioral health in this article), particularly in the wake of the coronavirus disease 2019 global pandemic. Impacts of pandemic on socialization, access to social services, family income, and physical health have negatively impacted youth mental health, leading to twice the volume of reported anxiety and depressive symptoms

[a] MetroHealth Medical Center, Case Western Reserve University School of Medicine, 2500 MetroHealth Drive, Cleveland, OH 44019, USA; [b] Miami University, 90 North Patterson Avenue, Oxford, OH 45056, USA; [c] Department of Psychological and Brain Sciences, Drexel University, 3141 Chestnut Street, Philadelphia, PA 19104, USA; [d] PolicyLab and the Center for Pediatric Clinical Effectiveness, Children's Hospital of Philadelphia (CHOP), 734 Schuylkill Avenue, Philadelphia, PA 19146, USA
* Corresponding author.
E-mail address: flaspopd@miamioh.edu

Pediatr Clin N Am 69 (2022) 709–723
https://doi.org/10.1016/j.pcl.2022.04.012
pediatric.theclinics.com
0031-3955/22/© 2022 Elsevier Inc. All rights reserved.

among youth in the United States.[2] To address high rates of depressive, anxious, and other distressing symptoms among youth, efforts to integrate behavioral health care and promotion into existing services have become popular strategies for increasing access to assessment and treatment. Pediatric primary care (PPC) and schools are 2 settings in which considerable research and practice have focused on this integration. Because these contexts differ considerably, professionals working in these settings have developed unique perspectives, research, and practices for integrating behavioral health care into daily activities. Considering these different perspectives may allow these 2 fields to learn from each other. Integrated school mental health (SMH) research, for example, places heavy emphasis on (1) effective interdisciplinary teamwork and (2) provision of services across tiers including "upstream" population-based prevention and promotion designed to meet their population's specific needs. "Upstream" services serve to promote wellness and prevent problems, rather than provide responsive treatment to problems that have already developed. This article argues that these 2 concepts from SMH have an opportunity for application in integrated PPC settings. Brief descriptions are provided for integrated behavioral health services in PPC and school settings. Next, 2 key concepts from SMH are detailed and suggestions are provided for application in integrated PPC settings.

INTEGRATED BEHAVIORAL HEALTH IN PEDIATRIC PRIMARY CARE SETTINGS

Integrating behavioral and medical care leads to positive outcomes for patients and providers. For patients, integrated care improves screening, identification, and intervention for developmental, behavioral, and mental health problems (eg, depression,[3] autism[4]), particularly for underserved patients who may otherwise have difficulty accessing behavioral health services.[4] Patients and caregivers report overall satisfaction with receiving integrated care and in fact report preferring to receive behavioral health intervention during routine medical visits.[5] Such treatment improves mental health outcomes across a variety of psychological disorders and is cost effective.[6] For primary care providers, integrated care reduces burnout and is linked to higher personal accomplishment and lower depersonalization.[7]

The benefits of integrated PPC are critical in the current climate where pediatric mental and behavioral health concerns are increasing[1,2] and factors such as stigma and lack of available mental health providers continue to limit access to treatment.[8,9] However, barriers to implementing integrated PPC exist, resulting in inconsistent use of integrated services both between and within primary care offices.[10] The current PPC model was not initially designed to address behavioral health. Therefore, many PPC offices lack the physical space needed for collocated services[11] as well as scheduling flexibility that allows for same day behavioral consultations or weekly or monthly appointments for ongoing behavioral health treatment.[12] Systemic factors such as lack of training for integrated care, "fee for service" pay structure, limited insurance coverage[13,14] for behavioral health care, and ongoing social stigma[10] also disrupt effective implementation.

Overcoming these barriers and creating an integrated system requires concentrated effort from clinicians and support staff. Many PPC offices, especially those not connected with academic or medical centers, do not have the capacity to provide training and dedicated time for their staff to develop the interdisciplinary competencies needed to support an integrated system.[13,15] This often results in small shifts toward integration or "business as usual" that does not fully meet the comprehensive behavioral health needs of patients. Furthermore, in primary care settings, behavioral health care often mimics the medical model, emphasizing response and treatment of identified problems. Researchers and clinicians have identified the need for behavioral health care in these settings to take a public health approach, emphasizing behavioral wellness promotion and preventive strategies as well as response and treatment.[16–18] This "upstream" approach may help increase early intervention and reduce stigma.

INTEGRATED BEHAVIORAL HEALTH IN SCHOOL SETTINGS

Similar to the PPC setting, school systems have identified the need to address nonacademic barriers to learning and development, including students' mental and behavioral health.[19,20] SMH practices ask schools to implement many programs that are new and perhaps not cohesive with traditional education models. These practices include behavioral screening, employment of behavioral health staff, school-wide positive behavior promotion systems, and lessons specifically designed to promote positive social and emotional development. Successful integration of SMH has resulted in positive psychosocial and academic outcomes for students.[21–23] To guide schools in adopting these practices without overwhelming limited staff capacity and school resources, a wide variety of frameworks exist for directing integration of mental health supports in schools (although descriptions are outside of the scope of this article).[24] These frameworks vary in perspective and implementation process, but share key tenants.[25] For example, SMH frameworks recommend use of a network of interdisciplinary teams to extend capacity and share strategic and implementation responsibilities among multiple groups.[19,24,26–28] Efficient teams in SMH have strong interdisciplinary teaming procedures, ongoing training and professional development opportunities, and access to school, community, and student data that guide decision making. Use of these teams has been linked to sustained SMH implementation and positive outcomes for student achievement and mental health.[29–31]

SMH best practices also recommend organizing behavioral health efforts in multi-tiered systems of support (MTSS) that address needs among 3 levels or tiers: tier 1 (universal behavioral health promotion programs for all students), tier 2 (indicated intervention for groups of students with known risk), and tier 3 (targeted treatment of students with diagnosed behavioral need) supports. Use of this 3-tiered approach is consistent with public health frameworks and ecological systems models of health[32] because it prioritizes behavioral wellness for all students while providing tailored support to students based on their level of need.[32] SMH specifically prioritizes creating supports across tiers that fit with the student population's specific needs and context. Although SMH programs still face implementation and sustainability challenges, these key principles have helped schools integrate behavioral health practices while building staff capacity and school resources. These same principles may be used to help fill the research and practice gaps identified in integrated PPC settings.

BUILDING CAPACITY FOR INTERDISCIPLINARY TEAMWORK

Integrating behavioral health into PPC and school settings requires interdisciplinary professionals to work in roles that are different from and in addition to their traditional responsibilities. Often, interdisciplinary staff operate in silos within the same setting, competing for resources and duplicating services. Interdisciplinary teaming helps allocate resources more efficiently, leading to reduced workloads and staff burnout.[29–31,33] Poorly implemented interdisciplinary teams, however, can have the opposite impact where resources used by the process outweigh positive outcomes.[34–36] SMH's layered teams approach establishes communication and planning systems that help facilitate the integration of behavioral supports.

EFFECTIVE INTERDISCIPLINARY TEAMING
Layered Teams

SMH practices suggest that effective teaming relies on a system of multiple teams and effective team meeting practices. SMH literature recommends allocating strategic and implementation tasks across multiple interdisciplinary teams, an overarching strategic leadership team and implementation team specific to one program or goal.[22] The strategic team is composed of members representing all relevant stakeholder groups (including families and students) and is connected to personnel in administration who have decision-making authority within the school.[37,38] This team may include a school psychologist, school social worker, school counselor, school nurse, teaching representatives, community behavioral health partners, a district liaison, school administrator, and caregivers representing the school community. Student voice can be included through a student representative or through consistent outreach via student surveys or interviews. Inclusion of all relevant stakeholders allows the team to transcend disciplinary silos and ensure multiple priorities are pursued with a coherent plan. The strategic team drives the integration of behavioral health services in the school through pursuit of 5 goals[30,39]: (1) determine the behavioral health needs of the school community, (2) identify strategies to meet these needs and promote behavioral wellness, (3) design an implementation plan, (4) provide training and technical assistance needed for implementation, and (5) collect data to evaluate progress and process.

To carry out these goals, strategic teams form and work with implementation teams.[39] Implementation teams comprise various staff or community members, based on the goal they are designed to achieve. For example, if a school wants to provide tier 1 social emotional learning (SEL) lessons to all students, the implementation team may include teachers who conduct the lessons and the school psychologist who provides technical assistance and evaluates the SEL program. The strategic team ensures that those responsible for implementation receive proper training and ongoing technical assistance.[37] The strategic team also ensures the implementation responsibilities are feasible. If the SEL lessons take 20 minutes of class time weekly, for example, and an additional 30 minutes of teacher time to prepare for the lessons, the strategic team must decide how to shift teachers' responsibilities or schedules to account for this time commitment. As the implementation team carries out tasks for the new program, they collect feedback and data related to the process (implementation) and progress (student outcomes). These data are reviewed by the strategic team to guide program progress.[37,39]

Team Practices

In addition to this teaming structure, SMH literature has identified meeting practices that impact the team's effectiveness, outputs, and morale of members. Each team member should have a clearly defined role on the team.[30] Important roles include a team leader, note-taker, data manager, and external communication manager. The team needs a shared virtual space where meeting agendas and documents are stored and easily accessible for all members.[30,39] The materials should include documentation of team mission, goals, decisions, and member roles and responsibilities. The team leader or note-taker sends an agenda to the team no less than 2 business days before the team meeting, allowing members to prepare and review relevant data before the team meeting so the meeting time is reserved for decision making. Finally, efficient teams agree upon communication practices for between-meeting communication,[30] including e-mail, phone calls, or other electronic tools based on the organizational culture and team preferences. These clear roles, meeting procedures, and avenues for communication enable efficiency by allowing teams to focus meeting time on pursuing their goals rather than managing teaming.

TRAINING AND PROFESSIONAL DEVELOPMENT

To implement these teaming processes, members require training and ongoing professional development. Often, professionals are asked to join a team or work with interdisciplinary staff without prior training on successful approaches to these processes. Providing a team with training on efficient meeting processes and evidence-based problem-solving methods can help the team be more efficient, solution-focused, and lead to higher rates of implementation, thereby improving student outcomes.[30] The Team-Initiated Problem Solving training has shown fidelity in helping teams increase their meeting and problem-solving skills on interdisciplinary SMH teams.[40–42] Involvement in learning communities with other similar teams also has shown promise in increasing teams' capacity and readiness for interdisciplinary teaming.[43] In addition to training for teaming, successful SMH relies on training that covers topics related to behavioral health. Many educational staff members have little training outside of their own discipline.[44] This little training may lead to professionals having different understanding of student behavior, evidence-based responses, and terminology. Professional development that provides learning on interdisciplinary topics relevant to team goals can help improve team members' knowledge and increase effective integration of behavioral health care.[44] A combination of initial training and ongoing coaching or technical assistance is needed to build and sustain team capacity.[30]

BUILDING CAPACITY THROUGH INTERDISCIPLINARY TEAMING: APPLICATION IN INTEGRATED PEDIATRIC PRIMARY CARE

In integrated PPC literature, few examples of layered teams have been described. An exception is the integrated behavioral health model developed based on the integrated practice assessment tool (IPAT) as described by Herbst and colleagues.[45] The IPAT model incorporates 4 elements to establish robust integrated PPC including clear mission and vision, universal prevention services, continuous quality improvement, and practice and systems transformation. This model shows promise[45] but has not yet been widely disseminated, particularly in PPC offices without resources supported by an academic medical center. Supporting this model through adoption of SMH teaming resources may help with dissemination and scale-up of the model. Related to training for integrated services, a wide range of activities have been described, such as shadowing, self-made manuals, allocation of professional development time, consultation, and external training.[15] However, there is limited evidence connecting these activities to increased capacity for integrated PPC or to patient outcomes. Several articles have described efficient coordinating operations for integrated PPC such as developing strong communication routes,[46] common goals between disciplines,[15] and use of an ethical acculturation model to prepare psychologists to work in integrated PPC.[47] In addition, most training emphasizes "fitting" psychologists into the medical setting rather than expanding the skill sets of professionals in both areas to pursue integrated work. These strategies have not been reported on in the context of teams facilitating implementation of integrated PPC.

Evidence-based SMH teaming processes may require adaptation to meet the needs of integrated PPC settings. **Table 1** outlines suggested adaptations, providing a

Table 1
Application of interdisciplinary teaming principles in integrated pediatric primary care

Teaming Component	Definition	Suggestions for Integrated PPC
Layered teaming: Strategic Leadership Team	Composed of representatives from all relevant stakeholders who have capacity to attend monthly or bimonthly meetings and dedicate approximately 2 additional hours per week to team activities	Team may include clinical staff (primary care provider, nurse, psychologist, and so on), administrative staff, family liaison, patient advocate, community partners (ie, social services, partnered medical center, local hospital) To ensure members have capacity, may need to adjust case load or job responsibilities to include strategic team activities
Layered teaming: Implementation Team	Composed of staff relevant to implementation goals, created when implementation is needed	If a PPC office identifies the need for parent education on preventing high blood lead levels, for example, the implementation team may include clinicians running a parent education seminar, and administrative staff for scheduling and preparation. The lead prevention team is responsible for identifying parents at need from provider referrals, conducting seminars, and collecting evaluation data. If needed, strategic team organizes office space, time in clinicians' schedules, and relevant training
Layered teaming: effective team processes	Evidence-based strategies that improve efficiency of team meetings, including clear roles, meeting agendas, shared space for documentation, communication strategies	In initial meetings, members determine roles that may be based on competencies related to their job or volunteers for positions such as leader, note-taker, and data analyst. Team determines meeting times and schedules and creates shared expectations for documentation, communication, and preparation for meetings

| Training and professional development: training to team | Training and professional development focused on building capacity for effective team strategies and working in an interdisciplinary setting | TIPS training has an evidence-base in SMH. Use of TIPS to establish meeting foundations and decision-making skills within teams may be applicable to integrated PPC |
| Training and professional development: training for interdisciplinary content | Training and professional development focused on specific topics related to integrated care | Examples may include evidence-based treatment for healthy sleep in integrated PPC, theories on origins of behavior from various disciplines |

Abbreviation: TIPS, team-initiated problem solving.

definition from SMH, and then proposing steps that may allow them to be adopted to fill implementation gaps in integrated PPC.

POPULATION-BASED PREVENTION AND INTERVENTION

Established SMH teams work to address behavioral health in schools at individual and aggregate community levels, consistent with public health, ecological systems, and MTSS frameworks. Within an MTSS framework, schools seek to provide preventive or behavioral wellness-promoting care to all students, targeted support to at-risk students, and direct intervention to students with an identified behavioral health need.[48] These multiple tiers of support are seen across social services and health care fields. SMH places priority on using student and community data to inform the types of universal, targeted, and directed interventions the school will provide.[30] This process includes data collection (or identification of available data), analysis of data in aggregate to understand population context, and use of findings to inform prevention, promotion, and intervention strategies.[49] In SMH, these processes are carried out by the strategic leadership team, relevant to strategic team goals 1 and 2 (described earlier).

The strategic team conducts a needs assessment of the community, identifying available data that are relevant to student behavioral well-being and making a plan to gather additional data as needed.[30,49–51] First, the team may identify data from school records. These data may include information on student achievement, student demographic data, number of students accessing resources such as free and reduced lunch, and office disciplinary referrals. The data also include information regarding the number and type of Individualized Education Plans and 504 Accommodations the school has in place for students. Schools also may be conducting universal screening of student behavioral symptoms (such as anxiety, inattention, hyperactivity, or depression). Although the screening itself may be part of a tier 1 universal approach to early identification of students needing tier 2 or tier 3 services, the data collected from these screenings can further inform the school's strategic behavioral health plan.

In addition to data available at the school level, the team's plan can be strengthened if informed by caregiver perspectives and information about students' community context.[30,49] In reaching out to caregivers, a strategic team may choose to send electronic or mail surveys, interview caregivers, conduct focus groups, or use a combination of these methods. Within these surveys or meetings, the strategic team seeks to learn about caregiver concerns regarding student behavior, at-home stressors, barriers to communication between caregivers and the school, and the priorities of caregivers in the community. In addition to caregiver-provided information, many counties or school districts have publicly available online databases that provide socioeconomic data about people living in that area.

Once these data are identified and collected, the strategic team's data analyst can review aggregate summaries of the information to look for patterns of behavioral health strengths and concerns and to identify contextual factors that facilitate these patterns. By understanding the community context, schools can be more aware of their students' needs and also be better prepared to choose services that are feasible given students' and families' contexts.[30] For example, a district that is located next to a large, industrial employer that hires many local employees to work first, second, or third shift may be able to infer that their students' caregivers are not regularly available at the same time. This inference could inform the strategic team that they need to offer social or caregiver activities at varying times to ensure caregivers working any shift have opportunities to participate.

The team may use various schedules to gather these data annually or at rolling times to inform their strategy over time. The universal, targeted, and directed treatment a school offers can then be chosen to specifically address the needs identified by reviewing the aggregate data, ensuring that services are specific to the student population's needs. This allows the school to be more proactive and efficient in providing specific services relevant to community needs versus providing generic behavioral health promotion or targeted small groups that are not based in the community context.

Population-Based Prevention and Intervention: Application in Integrated Pediatric Primary Care

In integrated PPC, there have been calls for using more population-based care practices.[52] PPC offices do use public health models that emphasize promotion, prevention, and treatment. Much of the prevention and promotion (tier one approaches) in PPC, however, are focused on universal screening procedures[53,54] and caregiver education.[12,55] The current literature reports primarily on the use of universal screening as a way for PPC providers to identify patients with behavioral concerns and connect them to intervention.[53,54] Although this is an important piece of behavioral health care, there are few reports of providers reviewing patient screeners in aggregate to learn more about patterns of need across their patient population. Similarly, there are few reports of PPC offices gathering community or caregiver information to identify and respond to specific behavioral health risks, strengths, and needs of their patient population. An exception exists in Herbst and colleagues'[45] application of the IPAT model in a PPC supported by an academic medical center. Widespread application of this population-based needs assessment to inform services provided has not been reported on in the literature.

There are evidence-based models for providing integrated tier 2 and tier 3 interventions in integrated PPC settings for specific behavioral disorders such as depression,[56] mood disorders,[56,57] and attention-deficit/hyperactivity disorder.[13] Although it may be ideal to train clinicians in each of these treatment modalities, providing or attending specific training for each of these models may overwhelm capacity. If an integrated PPC office is able to identify which treatment may be most relevant to their patient population, they may be able to prioritize that training first and meet a larger share of patient need. Similarly, behavioral health promotion and caregiver education practices can be tailored to the community resources and challenges experienced most frequently by their population while balancing readiness to respond to the variety of needs that arise among their patients. **Table 2** summarizes SMH's use of aggregate data to support population-based care and provides suggested adaptations or use in integrated PPC.

SUMMARY AND FUTURE DIRECTIONS

School and PPC settings have separately worked to integrate behavioral health care and promotion into their daily activities. As the fields have developed, so have new opportunities to learn from integration and capacity-building strategies. Integrated PPC shows promise but encounters barriers in implementation. The authors here propose that learning from SMH may be helpful for overcoming implementation barriers in integrated PPC. The establishment and training of layered teams as well as a focus on population-centered data and health promotion may enable integrated PPC settings to establish an "upstream" approach that more comprehensively supports behavioral wellness. Although perhaps promising, it is acknowledged that adopting these

Table 2
Application of population-based planning in integrated pediatric primary care

Population-Based Component	Definition	Suggestions for Integrated PPC
Data collection: existing data	Identifying information that is available from current processes relevant to behavioral health	• Intake demographic information • Insurance policy • Diagnoses (types, counts) • Prior treatment
Data collection: screeners	Short questionnaires given to families to identify areas of symptoms, risk, or need	Examples include ACEs,[58] SDQ,[59] RCADS,[60] PHQ-9,[61] CES-DC,[62] PSC-17[63]
Data collection: family information	Collecting information (existing or new) about family perceptions of children's behavioral development, needs, and impacting family or community factors	Questionnaires provided to families or inviting families to give feedback via interviews or focus groups upon check-in Strategic team may administer questions to interested families and record responses
Data collection: community context	Identifying existing information about community socioeconomic context, protective factors and resources, risk factors	Members of the strategic team review publicly available data to understand prominent protective and risk factors in the community that may impact child development and behavioral health
Data analysis	Strategic team (or data analyst) reviews data in aggregate, looking for patterns across the full population or within demographic groups. In the review with an interdisciplinary team, seeks to understand how community factors are connected to these patterns	Strategic team reviews patient diagnoses, demographics, common symptoms, family factors, and community risks and strengths. Looks for patterns between diagnoses or higher than expected symptoms that may indicate a community-specific need
Application of aggregate data	Strategic team reviews aggregate data trends and identifies promotion or treatment efforts that meet these needs	Conduct literature review to understand what evidence-based prevention, promotion, or intervention practices match population needs and context. Choose promotion practices and interventions that target population-specific needs to use resources efficiently. Create an implementation plan that fits staff capacity. Provide training and technical assistance as needed to implement population-specific programs

Abbreviations: ACEs, Adverse Childhood Experiences Questionnaire[58]; SDQ, strengths & difficulties questionnaire[59]; RCADS, revised child anxiety and depression scale[60]; PHQ-9, patient health questionnaire-9[61]; CES-DC, Center for Epidemiologic Studies Depression Scale for Children[62]; PSC-17, Pediatric Symptom Checklist.[63]

practices would not be without challenge and would require transformation of the current systems. Further research should explore the practicality and impact of adapting and adopting SMH principles of effective interdisciplinary teaming and "upstream" population-based prevention and intervention planning in integrated PPC contexts.

CLINICS CARE POINTS

- Create a patient registry of all patients seen by the pediatric practice; this could be done manually as each provider sees patients, or providers could use the tools built into electronic health records to automatically generate their patient registry. Creating a patient registry would help providers identify trends in patient presentation, screening measure results, and patient needs.

- When integrating behavioral health and medical care, consider using the layered teams approach by creating a strategic team and an implementation team (as described in this article). Consider including professionals from administration, billing/records, nursing, environmental services, and graduate medical education (if applicable), as well as patient and family representatives. The integrated practice should not consist of only providers.

- Advocate for protected provider time to allow for team meetings and reflection, data analyses, and quality improvement.

- Balance the needs to (1) provide care for each presenting problem, (2) provide preventative services, and (3) provide population health interventions based on the needs of the broader community. With the strategic team, explore alternative funding sources (such as grants) and billing structures (such as a patient-centered medical home) to support each layer of care.

DISCLOSURE

The authors have nothing to disclose.

REFERENCES

1. Reinfert M, Fritze D, Nguyen T. The state of mental health in America 2022. Alexandria, VA: Mental Health America; 2021.
2. Office of the Surgeon General (OSG). Protecting youth mental health: the U.S. surgeon general's advisory [Internet]. Washington, DC: US Department of Health and Human Services; 2021.
3. Farley AM, Gallop RJ, Brooks ES, et al. Identification and management of adolescent depression in a large pediatric care network. J Dev Behav Pediatr 2020; 41(2):85–94.
4. Hine JF, Allin J, Allman A, et al. Increasing access to Autism Spectrum Disorder diagnostic consultation in rural and underserved communities: Streamlined evaluation within primary care. J Dev Behav Pediatr 2020;41(1):16–22.
5. Riley AR, Wlaker BL, Wilson AC, et al. Parents' consumer preferences for early childhood behavioral intervention in primary care. J Dev Behav Pediatr 2019; 40(9):669–78.
6. Funk M. Integrating mental health into primary care: a global perspective. Geneva, Switzerland: World Health Organization; 2008.
7. Zubatsky M, Pettinelli D, Salas J, et al. Associations between integrated care practice and burnout factors of primary care physicians. Fam Med 2018; 50(10):770–4.
8. McMillan JA, Land M Jr, Leslie LK. Pediatric residency education and the behavioral and mental health crisis: A call to action. Pediatrics 2017;139:e20162141.

9. Stein REK, Horwitz SM, Storfer-Isser A, et al. Do pediatricians think they are responsible for identification and management of child mental health problems? Results of the AAP Periodic Survey. Ambul Pediatr 2008;8:11–7.

10. Tamene M, Morris A, Feinberg E, et al. Using the quality improvement (QI) tool failure models and effects analysis (FMEA) to examine implementation barriers to common workflows in integrated pediatric care. Clin Pract Pediatr Psychol 2020;8(3):257–67.

11. Snider TC, Raglin Bignall WJ, Hostutler CA, et al. Development and implementation of a culturally tailored early childhood program in an integrated pediatric primary care practice. Clin Pract Pediatr Psychol 2020;8(3):288–97.

12. Wissow LS, Ginneken N, Chandna J, et al. Integrating children's mental health into primary care. Pediatr Clin North Am 2015;63(1):97–113.

13. Leslie LK, Weckerly J, Plemmons D, et al. Implementing the American Academic of Pediatrics attention-deficit/hyperactivity disorder diagnostic guidelines in primary care settings. Pediatrics 2004;114(1):129–40.

14. American Academy of Child and Adolescent Psychiatry Committee on Health Care Access and Economics Task Force on Mental Health. Improving mental health services in primary care: Reducing administrative and financial barriers to access and collaboration. Pediatrics 2009;123:1248–51.

15. Hall J, Cohen D, Davis M, et al. Preparing the workforce for behavioral health and primary care integration. J Fam Med 2015;28:S41–51.

16. McCabe MA, Leslie L, Counts N, et al. Pediatric integrated primary care as the foundation for healthy development across the lifespan. Clin Pract Pediatr Psychol 2020;8(3):278–87.

17. Lines MM, Riley AR. Introduction to the special issue on integrated pediatric primary care: Placing "how" in the context of now. Clin Pract Pediatr Psychol 2020; 8(3):211–6.

18. Anderson-Butcher E, Stetler EG, Middle T. A case for expanded school-community partnerships in support of positive youth development. Children & Schools 2006;28(3):155–63.

19. DeLoach KP, Dvorsky M, Miller E, et al. Mental health issues and students with emotional and behavioral disorders. Behav Disord 2012;23:129–55.

20. Weist MD, Eber L, Horner R, et al. Improving multi-tiered systems of support for students with "internalizing" emotional/behavioral problems. J Pos Behav Interv 2018;20(3):172–84.

21. National Research Council and Institute of Medicine. Preventing mental, emotional, and behavioral disorders among young people: progress and possibilities. Washington, DC: The National Academies Press; 2009. https://doi.org/10.17226/12480.

22. Durlak JA, Weissberg RP, Dymnicki AB, et al. The impact of enhancing students' social and emotional learning: A meta-analysis of school-based universal intervention. Child Dev 2011;82(1):405–32.

23. Sklad M, Diekstra R, Ritter MD, et al. Effectiveness of school-based universal social, emotional, and behavioral programs: Do they enhance students' development in the area of skill, behavior, and adjustment? Psychol Sch 2012;49(9):892–909.

24. National Center for School Mental Health. SMH framework and tool alignment guidance document. 2021:1-7. Available at: https://www.schoolmentalhealth.org/media/SOM/Microsites/NCSMH/Documents/Resources/SMH-Framework-and-Tool-Alignment-Guidance-Document-11.29.20.pdf. Accessed September 1, 2022.

25. Hoover S, Lever N, Sachdev N, et al. Advancing comprehensive school mental health: guidance from the field. Baltimore, MD: National Center for School Mental Health. University of Maryland School of Medicine; 2019.

26. Waxman R, Weist MD, Benson D. Toward collaboration in the growing education mental health interface. Clin Psychol Rev 1999;19:239–53.

27. Bronstein L. A model for interdisciplinary collaboration. Social Work 2003;48: 297–306.

28. Powers JD, Edwards JD, Blackman KF, et al. Key elements of a successful multi-system collaboration for school-based mental health: In-depth interviews with district and agency administrators. Urban Rev 2013;45:651–70.

29. Kovaleski JF, Tucker JA, Duffy DJ Jr, et al. School reform through instructional support: The Pennsylvania Initiative. Part I: The instructional support team (IST) [and] Part II: Instructional evaluation. Communique 1995;23(8).

30. Splett J, Perales K, Halliday-Boykins C, et al. Best of practices for teaming and collaboration in the interconnected systems framework. J Appl Sch Psychol 2017;33(4):347–68.

31. Weist MD. Fulfilling the promise of school-based mental health: Moving toward a public mental health promotion approach. J Abnorm Child Psychol 2005;33(6): 735–41.

32. McIntosh K, Chard DJ, Boland JB, et al. Demonstration of combined efforts in school-wide academic and behavioral systems and incidence of reading and behavioral challenges in early elementary grades. J Pos Beh Interv 2006;8(3): 146–54.

33. Algozzine B, Newton JS, Horner RH, et al. Development and technical characteristics of a team decision-making assessment tool: Decision observation, recording, and analysis (DORA). J Psychoeduc Assess 2012;30(3):237–49.

34. Doll B, Haack K, Kosse S, et al. The dilemma of pragmatics: Why schools don't use quality team consultation practices. J Educ Psychol Consult 2005;16:127–55.

35. Mellin EA, Weist MD. Exploring school mental health collaboration in an urban community: A social capital perspective. Sch Ment Health 2011;3:81–92.

36. Cummings JN, Kiesler S. Coordination costs and project outcomes in multi-university collaborations. Res Policy 2007;36(1):1620–34.

37. Freeman R, Miller D, Newcomer L. Integration of academic and behavioral MTSS at the district level using implementation science. Learn Disabilities 2015;15(13): 59–72.

38. OSEP Technical Assistance Center on Positive Behavioral Interventions and Supports. Positive behavioral interventions and supports (PBIS) implementation blueprint: Part 1 - foundations and supporting information. Eugene (OR): University of Oregon; 2015. Available at: www.pbis.org.

39. National Center for School Mental Health, School mental health quality guide: teaming, 2020, NCSMH, University of Maryland School of Medicine; Baltimore, MD.

40. Horner RH, Newton JS, Todd AW, et al. A randomized waitlist controlled analysis of team-initiated problem solving professional development and use. Behav Dis 2018;43(4):444–56.

41. Newton JS, Horner RH, Algozzine B, et al. A randomized wait-list controlled analysis of the implementation integrity of team-initiated problem solving process. J Sch Psychol 2020;50:421–41.

42. Todd AW, Horner RH, Newton JS, et al. Effects of team-initiated problem solving on decision making by schoolwide behavior support teams. J Appl Sch Psychol 2011;27(1):42–59.

43. Connors EH, Smith-Millman M, Bohnenkamp JH, et al. Can we move the needle on school mental health quality through systematic quality improvement collaboratives? Sch Ment Health 2020;12:478–92.

44. Anderson EM, Bronstein LR. Examining interdisciplinary collaboration within an expanded school mental health framework: A community-university initiative. Adv Sch Ment Health Promot 2012;5(1):23–37.

45. Herbst RB, McClure JM, Ammerman RT, et al. Four innovations: A robust integrated behavioral health program in pediatric care. Fam Syst Health 2020; 38(4):450–63.

46. O'Reilly P, Lee SH, O'Sullivan M, et al. Assessing the facilitators and barriers of interdisciplinary team working in primary care using normalisation process theory: An integrative review. PLoS One 2017;12(5). https://doi.org/10.1371/journal.pone.0177026.

47. Jaques-Leonard ML, Winnick JB, Chancey LP, et al. Small town living: Unique ethical challenges of rural pediatric integrated primary care. Clin Pract Pediatr Psychol 2020. https://doi.org/10.1037/cpp00000339.

48. Stein W, Hoagwood K, Cohn A. School psychology: A public health perspective: I. Prevention, populations, and systems change. J Sch Psychol 2003;41(1): 23–38.

49. McIntosh K. and Goodman S., Integrated multi-tiered systems of support: blending RTI and PBIS, 2016, Guilford Publications; New York, NY.

50. Barrett S., Eber L. and Weist M.D., Advancing education effectiveness: an interconnected systems framework for positive behavioral interventions and supports (PBIS) and school mental health, 2013, University of Oregon Press; Eugene, OR.

51. Sugai G, Horner RH. Responsiveness-to-intervention and school-wide positive behavior supports: Integration of multi-tiered system approaches. Exceptionality: Spec Educ J 2009;17(4):223–37.

52. McDaniel H, Schiele B, Taylor LK, et al. Strengthening the components and processes of family involvement in school mental health. In: Weist M, Lever C, Bradshaw C, et al, editors. Handbook of school mental health: research, training, practice, and policy. 2nd edition. Boston, MA: Springer; 2014. p. 195–208.

53. Hourigan SE, Southam-Gerow MA, Quinoa AM. Emotional and behavioral problems in an urban pediatric primary care setting. Child Psychiatry Hum Dev 2015;46:289–99.

54. Burkhart K, Asogwa K, Muzaffar N, et al. Pediatric integrated care models: A systematic review. Clin Pediatr 2020;59(2):148–253.

55. Woods-Jaeger B, Thompson JE, Foye-Fletcher, et al. Parent engagement in an integrated care intervention to prevent toxic stress. Clin Pract Pediatr Psychol 2020;8(3):298–303.

56. Zuckerbrot RA, Cheung A, Jensen PS, et al. Guidelines for adolescent depression in primary care (GLAD-PC): Part I. Practice preparation, identification, assessment, and initial management. Pediatr 2018;141(3). https://doi.org/10.1542/peds.2017-4081.

57. Gerrity M. Evolving models of behavioral health integration: evidence update 2010-2015. 2016. Available at: https://www.milbank.org/publications/evolving-models-of-behavioral-health-integration-evidenceupdate-2010-2015/.

58. Felitti VJ, Anda RF, Nordenberg D, et al. Relationship of childhood abuse and household dysfunction to many of the leading causes of death in adults: the Adverse Childhood Experiences (ACE) study. Am J Prev Med 1998;14(4):245–58.

59. Goodman R. The strengths and difficulties questionnaire: A research note. J Child Psychol Pscychiatry 1997;38:581–6.

60. Chorpita BF, Yim L, Moffitt C, et al. Assessment of symptoms of DSM-IV anxiety and depression in children: a revised child anxiety and depression scale. Behav Res Ther 2000;38:835–55.
61. Kroenke K, Spitzer RL, Williams JB. The PHQ-9: validity of a brief depression severity measure. J Gen Intern Med 2001;16(9):606–13.
62. Weissman MM, Orvaschel H, Padian N. Children's symptoms and social functioning self-report scales: Comparison of mothers' and children's' reports. J Nerv Ment Disord 1980;168(12):736–40.
63. Murphy JM, Bergmann P, Chiang C, et al. The PSC-17: Subscale scores, reliability, and factor structure in a new national sample. Pediatrics 2016;138(3). https://doi.org/10.1542/peds.2016-0038.

Advancing School Behavioral Health at Multiple Levels of Scale

Mark D. Weist, PhD[a],*, Kristen Figas, EdS[a], Kelly Stern, MA[b,c],
John Terry, PhD[a], Erin Scherder, EdS[a], Darien Collins, BA[a],
Taylor Davis, EdS[a], Robert Stevens, PhD[a]

KEYWORDS

- Positive behavioral interventions and supports • Multitiered systems of support
- Interconnected systems framework • School behavioral health
- Collaborative partnerships • Communities of practice

KEY POINTS

- Integrating school behavioral health within multitiered systems of supports expands service accessibility to meet the growing behavioral health needs of children and youth.
- Successful integration requires collaborative partnerships that involve diverse stakeholders and effective teaming practices.
- Multilevel, bidirectional relationships (eg, between districts, states, and regions) improve coordination across systems and facilitate implementation at scale.
- Implementation support, including training and coaching, underlies the successful application of evidence-based practices and data-based decision-making within school behavioral health.

INTRODUCTION

Before COVID-19, approximately one in six children and youth in the United States had a diagnosable mental health condition, with only half of those children receiving treatment.[1] The shuttering of school buildings and prolonged interruption of typical schooling in response to COVID-19 has increased the strain on children and families, intensifying behavioral health concerns and underscoring the need for expanded behavioral health services.[2–4] Schools are the primary context in which children receive such services,[5] yet many schools struggle to meet the social-emotional and behavioral needs of students owing to provider shortages, undeveloped partnerships, and lack of capacity, policy, and funding support.[6–8] The ever-growing need for

[a] Department of Psychology, University of South Carolina, Barnwell College, 1512 Pendleton Street, Columbia, SC 29208, USA; [b] West Hawaii Complex Area, Hawaii School District; [c] Kealakehe High School – SBBH Office, 74-5000 Puohulihuli Street, Kalua-Kona, HI 96740, USA
* Corresponding author.
E-mail address: weist@sc.edu

Pediatr Clin N Am 69 (2022) 725–737
https://doi.org/10.1016/j.pcl.2022.04.004
0031-3955/22/© 2022 Elsevier Inc. All rights reserved.

pediatric.theclinics.com

behavioral health services for children, youth, and families underscores the necessity of streamlining services and integrating systems to improve efficiency, accessibility, and outcomes.

Multitiered System of Supports

The past 2 decades have seen the development of frameworks delineating a continuum of services for meeting the social-emotional and behavioral needs of children and youth. Multitiered system of supports (MTSS) represents one such framework designed to improve the implementation of school-based services across various levels of need. MTSS is an umbrella framework that structures the utilization of data and resources to inform prevention and intervention across three tiers—universal or school-wide approaches (Tier 1), targeted intervention for some students requiring additional support (Tier 2), and intensive intervention for those with more significant social-emotional, behavioral, and academic needs (Tier 3). Rather than focusing on a particular program or intervention, MTSS emphasizes a set of common practices that underlie effective implementation to promote positive outcomes. These practices are best articulated through the Positive Behavioral Interventions and Supports (PBIS) framework (see www.pbis.org/).[9]

PBIS is a well-established MTSS framework implemented widely in schools across the nation.[10] From its inception, the fundamental tenets of PBIS have included a systems perspective, teaming, data-based decision-making, implementation of evidence-based practices (EBPs), training and coaching to support implementation, aligning EBPs across tiers, and refining and improving them through ongoing progress monitoring.[9] When implemented with fidelity, PBIS has yielded a range of positive outcomes, including reductions in problem behavior and improvements in overall mental health and academic achievement of students and improvements in adult perceptions of school safety and organizational health.[11–14] However, PBIS has encountered implementation challenges at Tiers 2 and 3 and has limitations for addressing "internalizing" problems in students, such as anxiety, depression, and trauma-related issues.[15,16]

School Behavioral Health

Growing alongside PBIS, the school mental health movement historically focused on situating clinicians within schools to enhance the accessibility of mental health treatment.[17] Although school mental health has been demonstrated to increase access and consistency of mental health care and improve social-emotional and behavioral functioning of youth,[18,19] failing to integrate with schools' broader prevention and intervention frameworks ultimately limits the reach of this approach.

The Interconnected Systems Framework (ISF) for PBIS and school mental health is a conceptual framework for integrating these two approaches toward enhanced efficiency and outcomes.[15] We use the term school behavioral health (SBH) to refer to this more integrated approach. The ISF builds on the PBIS tradition by incorporating several critical elements that support effective PBIS and school mental health integration, such as effective partnerships and teaming practices, data-driven decision-making, enhanced screening of students' social-emotional and behavioral functioning, progress monitoring, outcome evaluation, data-driven intervention selection, implementation, and refinement, and ongoing implementation support. Greater depth in programming is also enabled across tiers as the behavioral health and education systems work together in a complementary manner.[15,20] The development and scaling of the ISF have been supported by the National Center on PBIS, with background information and a conceptual framework for it found at https://www.pbis.org/mental-health-social-emotional-well-being.

Critical Components of School Behavioral Health

Effective partnerships within SBH require diverse stakeholder involvement, representing families, children, and youth, school personnel (eg, teachers, administrators, school counselors, social workers, psychologists, and so forth), and staff and leaders from youth-serving community organizations.[15] SBH facilitates cross-system collaboration (eg, education, behavioral health, juvenile justice, and so forth) to provide a more extensive and integrated continuum of services.[16] Interdisciplinary partnerships increase efficiency by reducing the duplication of efforts and maximizing resources to circumvent implementation barriers.[15,21] Stakeholders comprise teams at multiple levels to support SBH implementation. State leadership teams are dedicated to sustaining and scaling the program by providing policy support, funding, technical assistance, and analyzing state-level data to guide implementation.[21] District-community leadership teams coordinate policy and funding and allocate resources at the district and school levels, whereas teams in individual schools are responsible for implementing practices to promote positive social-emotional, behavioral, and academic functioning.[21]

Data-based decision-making refers to the collaborative process of collecting, analyzing, and using data to guide intervention planning, implementation, and refinement. To better understand the context between social-emotional and behavioral needs and SBH implementation, the ISF promotes incorporating traditional sources of school-based data (eg, attendance, grades, and discipline) with community data (eg, on poverty, homelessness, violence, substance use).[15] Screening, progress monitoring, and outcome evaluation are integral to this process. Screening enables early identification, whereas progress monitoring and outcome evaluation equip teams to adjust interventions to maximize fit and gauge implementation fidelity.[15,16]

Within SBH, the effective implementation of EBPs is foundational, and their selection, implementation, and refinement occur within the team-based problem-solving process. Based on data and knowledge of the local context, teams select EBPs that can be aligned across tiers to facilitate effective implementation, tailor programming to varying levels of student needs, and promote coherence in the prevention to intervention continuum.[16] Tier 1 EBPs include positive behavior supports (eg, teaching, practicing, and reinforcing expected behavior) and social-emotional learning curricula, such as Second Step[22] or the Incredible Years,[23] which provide explicit instruction, guided practice, and reinforcement of target skills like social skills and emotional and behavioral regulation skills. Similarly, Tiers 2 and 3 EBPs, such as Check-in/Check-out[24] to support expected behavior, Coping Cat[25] for children with anxiety, or ACTION[26] for depressed youth, have common elements. Tiers 2 and 3 EBPs often target family or environmental risk factors, antecedents and consequences of behavior, and intrapersonal (cognitive or affective) processes by teaching skill-building to students, reinforcing new skills, and providing psychoeducation to children and their families. However, many schools encounter challenges implementing EBPs, and research suggests that EBPs are unlikely to achieve desired outcomes without implementation support.[27] The ISF promotes a team-based approach to professional development that combines training, coaching, and performance feedback to build knowledge and skills.[15]

The remainder of this article illustrates these critical components of SBH across multiple levels of scale, with implications for collaboration with health care systems. In the following, we describe strategies to promote effective SBH at district, state, and regional levels.

EFFECTIVE SCHOOL BEHAVIORAL HEALTH AT THE DISTRICT LEVEL
Multitiered Systems of Support in the West Hawaii Complex Area

The West Hawaii Complex Area covers 25 schools, including 19 K-12 public schools and 6 charter schools. It is essential to have a framework that clearly defines the critical components of a system-wide process to coordinate activities in a district of this size. The West Hawaii MTSS framework (see https://docs.google.com/drawings/d/1vQ23NzmOnJV4hQTrBvxtCKJbtoprgUB3QGSVFZuGv_o/edit?usp=sharing) illustrates the implementation of various components across tiers.

This work in West Hawaii has been informed by PBIS,[9] the ISF,[15] experienced national leaders/researchers (eg, Diana Browning Wright, Clay Cook), the adoption of MTSS as a priority statewide initiative, and large federal grants supporting this work (eg, the Project Advancing Wellness and Resiliency in Education from the Substance Abuse and Mental Health Services Administration). In the following, we review core components of the Hawaii MTSS with emphasis on Beliefs, Partnerships, Data-Based Decision Making, EBPs (across Tiers 1–3), and Implementation Support.

Beliefs

MTSS implementation efforts are impacted by beliefs that can function as barriers and need to be addressed for effective implementation.[28] In the West Hawaii school district, this challenge is addressed through the administration of the Beliefs about Behavior Survey[29,30] to predict implementation challenges. This psychometrically sound measure is administered to teachers, administrators, student support staff, and paraprofessionals to help the district understand beliefs that promote positive program implementation such as those related to building positive relationships and genuine collaboration and being proactive in the identification and response to student needs. The Beliefs about Behavior Survey also identifies challenging beliefs such as overvaluing punitive approaches or the student issues are someone else's problem such as a behavioral health professional. Understanding prevailing beliefs across schools in a district enables tailoring professional development and implementation support toward shared responsibility, improved role clarification, and the adjustment of problematic policies (such as emphasis on punitive measures).

Partnerships

In the process of establishing an MTSS framework, the first order of work is to compose a team comprised of multiple stakeholders, such as administrators, general education teachers, special education teachers, school counselors, social workers, school psychologists, behavioral health service providers, educational assistant staff, community and agency stakeholders, students, and family members. Team composition may vary by level, as do the roles and responsibilities of the teams. Teams are flexible, and additional members, such as pediatricians or other health care providers, may contribute when their expertise is needed. Indeed, school nurses are already active members of school teams, providing expertise on typical development, healthy environments, connections to community health resources, and the implementation of individual student health plans.[31] Although pediatricians and other health care providers can provide similar consultative support, expanding partnerships with the health care sector offers broader benefits, such as enhancing cross-system collaboration to align services for youth in pursuit of enhanced social, emotional, behavioral, and academic outcomes.

Data-based decision-making

In West Hawaii, data-based decision-making takes shape through the Team-Based Decision-Making Process and the Student Support Process, which are depicted in the MTSS logic model referenced above. These processes function as the way school teams work proactively to address student needs by moving students through the tiers as they are matched to appropriate levels of support. The Team Decision-Making Process specifies critical team members, data sources, and programs and interventions by tier and illustrates the practices and collaborations that permeate the entire MTSS framework. The Student Support Process refers to the process by which teams use data to match students to intervention and monitor progress. Integrating health care providers with school teams offers opportunities to mutually enhance decision-making by systematizing the process through which knowledge is shared across sectors. For example, health care providers can relay relevant information on a child's medical background and development that is meaningful for educational decision-making while also receiving educational information that informs diagnostic decisions and treatment planning.

Evidence-based practices

The following illustrates some of the tools used in West Hawaii to select EBPs, support implementation, collect progress monitoring data, and refine practices over time. Additional information on West Hawaii MTSS and resources for each tier are accessible on the West Hawaii School-Based Behavioral Health Web site.[31]

Tier 1 practices. Tier 1 focuses on universal or school-wide support structures and programs. In West Hawaii, we use the Tiered Fidelity Inventory[32] to identify Tier 1 best practices and guide implementation efforts that can be measured and addressed. This free and downloadable implementation tool guides the evaluation and implementation of the critical components of PBIS. Tier 1 practices include selecting social–emotional learning programs, conducting universal social-emotional and behavioral screening, developing core PBIS processes, and providing consultation for school-wide crisis response. Implementation of Tier 1 practices, such as universal screening and social-emotional learning programs, is monitored through the Tiered Fidelity Inventory. At Tier 1, health care providers can consult on the selection of social–emotional learning curricula and universal screening tools that reflect the behavioral health needs of the community and integrate best practices in supporting the holistic development of youth. This collaboration might also open the opportunity for health care providers to use universal social-emotional and behavioral screening data to inform community health care services. For instance, understanding the priority concerns of the local youth population, as measured by school screeners, would enable health care providers to adapt their typical health care services in response, thus facilitating cross-system alignment.

Tier 2 practices. The goal of Tier 2 support is to identify and support students who present social-emotional and behavioral needs that require more than universal (Tier 1) programming to be successful. At Tier 2, teams use the Student Intervention Matching form[33] to streamline decision-making, thus allowing teams to focus on intervention fidelity and progress monitoring. The 18-item protocol facilitates matching students to Tier 2 interventions and has been shown to improve outcomes for students.[34] This form is accessible through the West Hawaii School-Based Behavioral Health site,[31] which includes information on evidence-based Tier 2 interventions and progress monitoring tools. Tier 2 teams support intervention implementation and regularly review progress monitoring data. At Tier 2, health care providers can contribute medical and developmental information to inform intervention selection while also receiving information on a child's educational needs and progress to inform their own diagnostic impressions, treatment, or referral to specialty medical services.

Tier 3 practices. At Tier 3, the focus is on individualized interventions. Tier 3 teams meet to review individual student data and develop intervention plans tailored to a student's particular needs. For example, this might involve individual counseling, behavior support plans, multiagency collaboration, crisis intervention, individual safety plans, and/or in-class support. In the West Hawaii MTSS model, these interventions often are selected from the PracticeWise system, a modular strategy for evidence-based mental and behavioral health intervention for youth and families.[35] Although various data sources may be used to monitor progress at this level, the Behavior Intervention Monitoring Assessment System[36] is commonly used to monitor the progress of students receiving counseling. At Tier 3, coordination between schools and health care providers acquires greater urgency. At this stage, school practitioners and health care providers can collaborate on psychoeducational evaluations to ensure a student's strengths and needs are examined, safety planning for students in acute crisis such as those experiencing suicidal ideation,[37] referral to specialty services, or reentry planning when students require acute psychiatric care for a period of time.

Implementation support
Implementation support is critical to ensure interventions are selected appropriately and implemented with fidelity. Districts can assist by providing training and coaching for ongoing support. The West Hawaii School-Based Behavioral Health team offers weekly behavior laboratories facilitated by practice area leaders to provide frequent consultative support to individuals and teams. Practice area leaders include a licensed clinical psychologist, board-certified behavior analyst, and coaches with specialized content knowledge (eg, MTSS, dialectical behavior therapy, de-escalation, universal screening). Additional support is provided to help role groups learn their role in intervention implementation. For example, teachers might need clarification on how to provide support at different tiers (eg, teaching class-wide social-emotional and behavioral expectations, reteaching expectations to a small group, and individualizing reminders for one or two students). Individuals with expertise in specific areas provide specialized support. For instance, a behavioral health professional might assist teams with using data to determine school-wide social-emotional and behavioral skills (Tier 1), assist with Tier 2 group interventions to reaffirm those skills, and incorporate those skills in treatment planning at Tier 3. Thus, toward building coherent and impactful programming, there is a strong emphasis on aligning programs across tiers, highlighting the national center on PBIS, which works closely with the Hawaii program (see https://www.pbis.org/resource/school-mental-health-quality-framework-and-tools-alignment-guide).

STATE-LEVEL STRATEGIES FOR ADVANCING SCHOOL BEHAVIORAL HEALTH
Behavioral Alliance of South Carolina

South Carolina (SC) has made substantial headway in advancing SBH by developing an innovative collaboration called the Behavioral Alliance of South Carolina (BASC).[38,39] BASC is a partnership between the SC Department of Education, Office of Special Education Services, and the Southeastern School Behavioral Health Community led by the SBH Team at the University of South Carolina that increases the capacity of school districts to support the social, emotional, behavioral, and academic functioning of students. Mirroring MTSS, BASC uses a multi-realm approach to structure activities across the state, focusing priorities in three realms. Realm I consists of the Southeastern School Behavioral Health Community annual conference and associated online resource repository. Targeted support is provided in Realm II through newsletters, training webinars, an online resource library, and virtual programs. Realm

III offers direct training and implementation support to districts. BASCs progress across dimensions of Partnerships, Data-based Decision Making (including screening and progress monitoring), and Implementation Support is reviewed in the following.

Partnerships

BASC approaches collaboration through a lens of identifying organizations and extant teams with similar missions to reduce siloed service delivery and duplication of effort. BASC integrates stakeholder involvement across SC, including the Office of Special Education Services, the SC Department of Mental Health, University of South Carolina Psychology Department and College of Education, Mid-Atlantic PBIS (https://midatlanticpbis.org/), Midwest PBIS (https://midwestpbis2.org/), and leaders from key youth service organizations.

The BASC State Leadership Team[21] coordinates operations and promotes the achievement of goals by providing consultative support to districts. The leadership team meets quarterly to discuss progress, engage in problem-solving, identify next steps, and create and supervise "community of practice" groups. Communities of practice are groups of professionals that collect to share knowledge and engage in collaborative problem-solving.[40] BASC supports the development of communities of practice, bringing together educators, administrators, and SBH practitioners to expand participants' knowledge and skills, encourage mutual support and problem-solving, and promote the sustainment of positive school changes. BASCs efforts to expand team membership and involve stakeholders from various state agencies have increased participation across the state. In response to COVID-19, BASC enhanced team effectiveness by providing virtual opportunities for collaboration among schools and youth-serving systems focused on improving programs for children and youth. Virtual meetings included focus groups, collaborative work time, and concept mapping to enhance teaming processes.

Data-based decision-making

BASC follows ISF recommendations for data-based decision-making at the state level.[15] BASC team leaders compile data supplied by school districts on previous initiatives, progress, and outcomes (eg, attendance, universal screening, nurse visits, office discipline referrals, suspensions, community partnerships, and so forth). Data are used to complete needs assessment to assist strategic planning on SBH improvement. This process includes reviewing the data sources districts use to assess student needs to identify gaps in existing data sources. As an example, this process has resulted in additional guidance on universal screening and the inclusion of community data on students' needs. BASC also supports quarterly and yearly routines for team-led data-based decision-making across the state. Walking alongside districts and with state leaders, BASC has facilitated root cause analysis problem-solving through a review of disproportionality data to identify schools/districts needing additional coaching and implementation support.

Screening. Conducting screening on students' social–emotional–behavioral functioning is a unique hurdle at the local and state levels. School personnel have reported experiencing more challenges with universal screening than other SBH elements. BASC responded to this need by issuing guidance on screening, including screening expectations that districts can tailor before implementation. BASC promotes the use of the Best Practices in Universal Social, Emotional, Behavioral Screening playbook,[41] which outlines expectations such as recommended type of screener, screening schedules, developing an implementation plan, integrating screening with other data sources, and sharing information.

Progress monitoring and outcome evaluation. BASC assesses progress monitoring data quarterly and outcome data yearly. The BASC progress monitoring process involves analyzing the number of children receiving services, implementation challenges, and implementation strengths. Conference, webinar, and technical assistance presentations to the BASC Leadership Team have highlighted exclusionary practices and disparities in attendance, school engagement, academic achievement, and school climate and functioning. The ISF-Implementation Inventory[42] was used before COVID-19 to assess fundamental elements of SBH implementation for performance monitoring, continuous process improvement, and outcome evaluation. BASC continues to use the ISF-Implementation Inventory as a coaching tool while allowing districts to choose other fidelity measures such as the Tiered Fidelity Inventory.[26] BASC provides coaching around selecting fidelity measures and integrated action planning following their use.

Implementation support at the state level

BASC provides implementation support for EBPs in prevention, small group intervention, social-emotional learning programs, and intensive interventions at the district and school levels. BASC has developed an e-manual on High Leverage Practices, an online resource library, and webinars featuring national researchers and SBH professionals. BASC offers training on brief evidence-based treatment modules focused on improving behavioral health literacy, associated with improved student functioning and reduced stigma/increased help-seeking.[43] During the initial days of COVID-19, BASC updated virtual platforms to give weekly mini skill-based webinars related to current events.

BASC also provides training and technical assistance for MTSS implementation. The BASC coaches and community partners promote bidirectional communication with districts to guide programming through co-coaching environments. School districts receive onsite support, remote training, and implementation help from BASC coaches. For example, BASC has supported the implementation of universal screening at the district level through webinars, checklists with pre-implementation guidance, and direct coaching to the school leadership team.

ADVANCING SCHOOL BEHAVIORAL HEALTH AT THE REGIONAL LEVEL

The previous section outlined lessons learned in advancing SBH through a multitiered perspective at district and state levels. At the state level, we see purposeful actions taken for effective teaming including diverse stakeholders, collecting and using data for decision-making, and implementation support through co-coaching and bidirectional communication.

Regional organizations support SBH efforts with some of the same action states use, but they have a broader view of building SBH capacity and expertise. Two prominent examples of regional organizations supporting SBH are the regional Mental Health Technology Transfer Centers, and the regional centers focused on effective MTSS such as the Mid-Atlantic PBIS Network, the Midwest PBIS Network, and the Southeastern School Behavioral Health Community. The Southeast Mental Health Technology Transfer Center (https://mhttcnetwork.org/) promotes the adoption of evidence-based mental health services and provides training and technical assistance to state SBH leaders in the region. Regional PBIS networks aim to develop the capacity of schools to address SBH and assist state departments of education and other state agencies with installation, fidelity, outcomes, and sustainability. The missions of these regional organizations are to provide support to state leaders, as opposed to direct support of school staff and students. The Mental Health Technology Transfer

Center and PBIS networks along with other regional efforts such as the National Quality Initiative from the School-Based Health Alliance assist states in identifying appropriate EBPs and in many cases provide evidence-based materials and train-the-trainer opportunities, including an emphasis on developing and sustaining effective SBH programs.

In addition to the formal regional efforts funded and supported by large national organizations, several grassroots organizations have been created through state SBH leaders to facilitate collaboration across a region. Two examples of these home-grown regional organizations are the Carolina Network for School Mental Health and the Southeastern School Behavioral Health Community. Both organizations have grown out of a "community of practice" that coalesced in their regions. The Carolina Network (www.carolinanetwork.org/) was conceptualized to enhance the awareness of school mental health initiatives near one another and facilitate productive collaborations within and between states, including clinical activities, empirical endeavors, policy development, and dissemination of EBP. The Southeastern School Behavioral Health Community (www.schoolbehavioralhealth.org/) focuses on advancing research, best practices, and policy on effective SBH programs that reflect the mental health system partnering with schools and linking with multitiered systems of support, such as PBIS. Both efforts are good examples of regional organizations that develop locally, without the formal connection and guidance from a large parent organization.

DISCUSSION

The movement toward a full continuum of behavioral health supports for students through SBH programs involving mental health system integration into schools' multitiered systems of support has grown progressively in recent years and is being further propelled by significantly elevated social–emotional and behavioral needs of children and youth associated with the COVID-19 pandemic and related severe societal stressors. SBH programs are growing throughout the United States and in other nations.[44] In this work, there is a strong emphasis on implementing the most effective programs and practices to improve students' social-emotional, behavioral, and academic functioning, including implementing EBPs, coaching, team functioning, aligning strategies across tiers, data-based decision-making, progress monitoring, and outcome evaluation.[9,15,16]

In this article, we describe the development of SBH at multiple levels of scale, including the school district, state, and regional levels. At each of these levels, there is an emphasis on building a community of practice,[37] paying purposeful attention to building and growing relationships with diverse stakeholders including educators, clinicians, families and youth, staff and leaders from other youth serving organizations (eg, child welfare, juvenile justice, primary care), policymakers and researchers.[45] There is an emphasis on leading by convening,[46] and as relationships develop, moving from discussion to dialogue, genuine collaboration, identification and utilization of expanded resources, and policy change. Through this work, social capital is developed, and this is associated with escalation in the pace of positive change.[47]

Under the umbrella of SBH, there are many opportunities for collaboration between schools and health care providers to streamline behavioral health services for youth. At Tier 1, partnerships between clinicians and schools provide an avenue for bidirectional knowledge transfer that benefits youth and families. In the context of consultation with school leadership teams or professional development, clinicians can offer guidance on best practices in behavioral health care and expand their knowledge of best practices in SBH. Beyond sharing expertise, this collaboration provides an opportunity for clinicians and SBH staff to bridge differences in language, diagnostic criteria, and treatment approaches that cause confusion for educators and families. At Tier 2, clinicians can collaborate with school teams on intervention planning, progress monitoring, and outcome evaluation to ensure alignment between school and behavioral health care services, thus reducing redundancy, improving decision-making, and clarifying messaging to families. Clinicians can engage in similar work at Tier 3, in addition to consulting with school teams to navigate referrals between education and health care systems and coordinating acute care and reentry planning.

There should also be a focus on metacognition, or thinking about thinking,[48] and considering if the processes are playing out most effectively within and across levels of scale. For example, is there an effective, interdisciplinary team at the school district level, including stakeholders reviewed above, who have expertise and authority to allocate resources for effective SBH within school buildings?[15] This involves horizontal collaboration among staff and stakeholders at district and building levels and vertical collaboration between these levels. The emphasis on metacognition would also include strategies to improve the effectiveness of all planning processes such as using validated tools to monitor and provide support to assure the fidelity of all practices within the MTSS.[32,35]

SUMMARY

The COVID-19 pandemic has further underscored the significance of comprehensive and proactive approaches, which support the holistic mental and behavioral wellness of our students, educators, and communities at large.[2–4] These strategies are best modeled through the application of effective SBH programming that includes diverse and vested stakeholders empowered with evidence-based, culturally relevant strategies, modeled in the ISF,[15] to promote positive social, emotional, behavioral, and academic outcomes. Critical to the success of SBH is enhanced implementation capacity achieved through prioritization of effective teaming, which highlights multiple levels of coordinated involvement including school, district, state, and regional levels of scale and leadership.

CLINICS CARE POINTS

- Essential to the effective integration of behavioral health system staff into a multitiered system of supports (MTSS) framework is their inclusion in professional development opportunities, which enhance their knowledge of the foundations and language of Positive Behavioral Interventions and Supports.

- Clinicians foster protective factors at Tier 1 through the provision of school level mental health trainings (foundational knowledge, protocols/procedures, best practice intervention strategies, function of behavior, and so forth.) which promote early identification and intervention, cohesive programming within the MTSS, and positive social, emotional, behavioral, and academic outcomes among students.

- Behavioral health staff from the behavioral health and education systems and educators emphasize interdisciplinary collaboration including families and enhance horizontal communication at building and district levels and vertical communication between these levels.

- Using clinicians as leaders and coaches across all three tiers of support of the MTSS expands their role beyond assessment and intervention and increases capacity for best practices at all tiers, resulting in better tailoring of supports and services to match student/family strengths and needs.

FUNDING STATEMENT

This publication was made possible in part by Grant Number T32-GM081740 from NIH-NIGMS. Its contents are solely the responsibility of the authors and do not necessarily represent the official views of the NIGMS or NIH.

DISCLOSURE

The authors have no conflicts of interest to disclose.

REFERENCES

1. Whitney DG, Peterson MD. US national and state-level prevalence of mental health disorders and disparities of mental health care use in children. JAMA Pediatr 2019;173(4):389–91.
2. Jones EA, Mitra AK, Bhuiyan AR. Impact of COVID-19 on mental health in adolescents: a systematic review. Int J Environ Res Public Health 2021;18(5):1–9.
3. Patrick SW, Henkhaus LE, Zickafoose JS, et al. Well-being of parents and children during the COVID-19 pandemic: a national survey. Pediatrics 2020; 146(4):1–8.
4. Verlenden JV, Pampati S, Rasberry CN, et al. Association of children's mode of school instruction with child and parent experiences and well-being during the COVID-19 Pandemic — COVID experiences survey, United States, October 8–November 13, 2020. MMWR Morb Mortal Wkly Rep 2021;70:369–76.
5. Juszczak L, Melinkovich P, Kapan D. Use of health and mental health services by adolescents across multiple delivery sites. J Adolesc Health 2003;32(6):108–18.
6. Eklund K, DeMarchena SL, Rossen E, et al. Examining the role of school psychologists as providers of mental and behavioral health services. Psychol Sch 2020; 57(4):489–501.
7. Oullette PM, Briscoe R, Tyson C. Parent-school and community partnerships in children's mental health: Networking challenges, dilemmas, and solutions. J Child Fam Stud 2004;13(2):295–308.
8. Stephan S, Hurwotz L, Paternite C, et al. Critical factors and strategies for advancing statewide school mental health policy and practice. Adv Sch Ment Health Promot 2010;3(3):48–58.
9. Sugai G, Horner RR. A promising approach for expanding and sustaining school-wide positive behavior support. Sch Psych Rev 2006;35(2):245–59.
10. OSEP Technical Assistance Center on Positive Behavioral Interventions and Supports. 2020. Available at: pbis.org. Accessed October 6, 2021.
11. Lee A, Gage N. Updating and expanding systematic reviews and meta-analyses on the effects of school-wide positive behavior interventions and supports. Psychol Sch 2020;47(4):783–804.
12. Cook CR, Frye M, Slemrod T, et al. An integrated approach to universal prevention: Independent and combined effects of PBIS and SEL on youths' mental health. Sch Psychol Q 2015;30(2):166–83.
13. Horner T, Sugai G, Smolkowski K, et al. A randomized control trial of school-wide positive behavior support in elementary schools. J Posit Behav Interv 2009;11: 133–44.
14. Bradshaw CP, Koth CW, Thornton LA, et al. Altering school climate through school-wide positive behavioral interventions and supports: Findings from a group-randomized effectiveness trial. Prev Sci 2009;10(2):100–15.

15. Eber L, Barrett S, Perales K, et al. Advancing education effectiveness: Interconnecting school mental health and school-wide PBIS, volume 2: an implementation guide. Center for Positive Behavior Interventions and Supports (funded by the Office of Special Education Programs, U.S. Department of Education). Eugene (OR): University of Oregon Press; 2020.

16. Weist MD, Eber L, Horner R, et al. Improving multitiered systems of support for students with "internalizing" emotional/behavioral problems. J Pos Behav Interv 2018;20(3):172–84.

17. Flaherty LT, Osher D. History of school-based mental health services in the United States. In: Weist MD, Evans SW, Lever NA, editors. Handbook of school mental health: advancing practice and research. New York: Springer; 2003. p. 11–22.

18. Atkins MS, Frazier SL, Birman D, et al. School-based mental health services for children living in high poverty urban communities. Adm Policy Ment Health 2006;33(2):146–59.

19. Ballard KL, Sander MA, Klimes-Dougan B. School-related and social-emotional outcomes of providing mental health services in schools. Community Ment Health J 2014;50:145–9.

20. Weist MD, Franke KB, Stevens RN. Advancing effective school behavioral health. In: Weist MD, Franke KB, Stevens RN, editors. School behavioral health: interconnecting comprehensive school mental health and positive behavior support. New York: Springer; 2020. p. 1–8.

21. Splett J, Perales K, Halliday-Boykins C, et al. Best practices for teaming and collaboration in the Interconnected Systems Framework. J Appl Sch Psychol 2017;33(4):347–68.

22. Frey KS, Hirchstein MK, Guzzo BA. Second step: Preventing aggression by promoting social competence. J Emot Behav Disord 2000;8(2):102–12.

23. Webster-Stratton C, Reid MJ. The Incredible Years parents, teachers, and children training series: A multifaceted treatment approach for young children with conduct problems. In: Weisz JR, Kazdin AE, editors. Evidence-based psychotherapies for children and adolescents. New York: Guilford Press; 2018. p. 122–41.

24. Todd AW, Campbell AL, Meyer GG, et al. The effects of a targeted intervention to reduce problem behaviors: Elementary school implementation of Check In–Check Out. J Posit Behav Interv 2008;10(11):46–55.

25. Kendall PC, Kedtke K. Cognitive-behavioral therapy for anxious children: therapist manual. 3rd ed. Ardmore: Workbook Publishing; 2006.

26. Stark KD, Streusand W, Arora P, et al. Childhood depression: The ACTION treatment program. In: Kendall PC, editor. Child and adolescent therapy. 4th ed. New York: Guilford Press; 2011. p. 190–233.

27. Sugai G, Horner R. Sustaining and scaling positive behavioral interventions and supports: Implementation drivers, outcomes, and considerations. Except Child 2020;86(2):120–36.

28. Cook CR, Lyon AR, Kubergovic D, et al. A supportive beliefs intervention to facilitate the implementation of evidence-based practices within a multi-tiered system of supports. Sch Ment Health 2015;7(1):49–60.

29. Wright DB, Cook CR. Beliefs about behavior –. 4th edition 2012. Available at: https://www.sjcoe.org/selparesources/tiers/Beliefs%20About%20Behavior%20_4th%20edition_%2030%20items.pdf. Accessed September 27, 2021.

30. Holmes BW, Sheetz A, Allison M, et al. Role of the school nurse in providing school health services. Pediatrics 2016;137(6):1–6.

31. West Hawaii School-Based Behavioral Health. 2021. Available at:https://sites. google.com/k12.hi.us/west-hawaii-sbbh/home. . Accessed on October 12, 2021.
32. Algozzine B, Barrett S, Eber L, et al. School-wide PBIS tiered fidelity inventory. OSEP Technical Assistance Center on Positive Behavioral Interventions and Supports. 2019. Available at: https://www.pbis.org/resource-type/assessments. Accessed September 27, 2021.
33. Cook CR. Student intervention matching form (SIM-form) [PDF]. 2011. Available at: https://sesccoop.org/wp-content/uploads/2015/12/Student-Intervention-Matching-Form.pdf.
34. Miller FB, Cook CR, Zhang Y. Initial development and evaluation of the student intervention matching (SIM) form. J Sch Psychol 2018;66:11–24.
35. PracticeWise LLC. Blue menu of evidence-based psychosocial interventions for youth. 2021. Available at: https://www.practicewise.com/portals/0/forms/Practice Wise_Blue_Menu_of_Evidence-Based_Interventions.pdf. Accessed September 27, 2021.
36. McDougal JL, Bardos AN, Meier ST. Behavior intervention monitoring assessment system 2. Torrance, CA: WPS Publishers; 2016.
37. Breslin K, Balaban J, Shubkin C. Adolescent suicide: What can pediatricians do? Curr Opin Pediatr 2020;32(4):595–600.
38. Franke K, Paton M, Weist M. Building policy support for school mental health in South Carolina. Sch Psych Rev 2020;50(1):110–21.
39. Shapiro C, Collins C, Parker J, et al. Coalescing investments in school mental health in South Carolina. Child Adol Ment Health 2020;25:150–6.
40. Wenger E, McDermott RA, Snyder W. Cultivating communities of practice: a guide to managing knowledge. Boston, MA: Harvard Business Press; 2002.
41. Romer N, von der Embse N, Eklund K, et al. Best practices in social, emotional, and behavioral screening: an implementation guide. 2020. Available at: https:// smhcollaborative.org/universalscreening/. Accessed September 27, 2021.
42. Splett JW, Perales K, Al-Khatib A, et al. Preliminary development and validation of the interconnected systems framework implementation inventory (ISF-II). Sch Psychol 2020;35(4):255–66.
43. Clauss-Ehlers C, Carpio MG, Weist MD. Mental health literacy: a strategy for global mental health promotion. Adol Psychia 2020;10(2):73–83.
44. Weist MD, Bruns E, Whitaker K, et al. School mental health promotion and intervention: Experiences from four nations. Sch Psychol Interntl 2017;38(4):343–62.
45. Weist MD, Collins D, Martinez S, et al. Furthering the advancement of school behavioral health in your community. In: Weist MD, Franke K, Stevens R, editors. School behavioral health: interconnecting comprehensive school mental health and positive behavior support. New York: Springer; 2020. p. 123–8.
46. Cashman J, Linehan P, Purcell L, et al. Leading by convening: a blueprint for authentic engagement. Alexandria, VA: National Association of State Directors of Special Education; 2014.
47. Mellin EA, Weist MD. Exploring school mental health collaboration in an urban community: A social capital perspective. Sch Ment Health 2011;3(2):81–92.
48. Dunlosky J, Metcalfe J. Metacognition: a textbook for cognitive, educational, life span & applied psychology. Washington, DC: Sage; 2009.

Synthesizing Adaptive Digital Bioethics to Guide the Use of Interactive Communication Technologies in Adolescent Behavioral Medicine
A Systematic Configurative Review

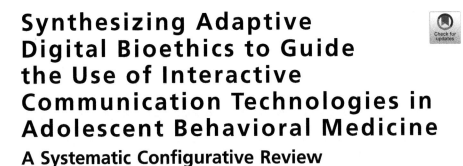

Simone J. Skeen, MA[a],*, Sara K. Shaw Green, MSW[b],
Amelia S. Knopf, PhD, MPH, RN[c]

KEYWORDS

- Digital bioethics • Interactive communication technologies • Autonomy
- Adolescence • Behavioral health

KEY POINTS

- The rapid pace with which digital tools evolve, are creatively reappropriated by young people, and integrated into clinical preventive services, requires innovative ethical frameworks to guide their use.
- The misuse of digital tools can exacerbate digitally mediated harms that stem from fundamental properties of interactive communication technologies. These harms include reputational damage, distress, and breaches of privacy.
- The use of digital outreach tools in human immunodeficiency virus (HIV) prevention science informs ethical safeguards applicable to their broader clinical use, with particular emphasis on protecting youth autonomy and privacy.
- Safeguards to mitigate against digitally mediated harms in the course of service/study interactions include knowledge of unique needs of youth subpopulations, integration of recurring digital safety assessments into clinical care, and caution regarding smartphone notifications.

[a] Department of Social, Behavioral, and Population Sciences, School of Public Health and Tropical Medicine, Tulane University, 1440 Canal Street, New Orleans, LA 70112, USA; [b] Center for Translational Behavioral Science, Florida State University, 2010 Levy Avenue, Research Building B, Suite B0266, Tallahassee, FL 32310, USA; [c] Community and Health Systems, Indiana University School of Nursing, 600 Barnhill Drive, NU W425, Indianapolis, IN 46220, USA
* Corresponding author.
E-mail address: sskeen@tulane.edu

Pediatr Clin N Am 69 (2022) 739–758
https://doi.org/10.1016/j.pcl.2022.04.006
0031-3955/22/© 2022 Elsevier Inc. All rights reserved.

INTRODUCTION

In 2018, 95% of teens in the United States aged 13–17 years owned or had access to a smartphone.[1] The ubiquity of smartphones has altered the social landscape of teens and provided new mechanisms for researchers and clinicians to interact with them. In 2015, the Health Resources and Services Administration's (HRSA's) HIV/AIDS Bureau launched the *Using Social Media to Improve Engagement, Retention, and Health Outcomes along the HIV Care Continuum Initiative*, supporting a range of HIV care providers in using smartphone- and social media-facilitated techniques to connect with adolescents and young adults (AYA).[2] This initiative is consistent with a broader trend toward integrating digital outreach tools into AYA-focused clinical preventive services.[3] In 2021 alone, the National Institutes of Health awarded more than $66 million to researchers using digitally networked interactive communication technologies (ICTs, typically smartphone-enabled, or "mobile") to intervene on and improve the health of AYA.[4] Use of ICTs is not limited to intervention delivery—they are also used to identify, recruit, and retain AYA in sociobehavioral and clinical studies.[5,6] ICTs can be understood in terms of emergent *affordances,* "those fundamental properties that determine just how the thing could possibly be used,"[7,8] which are relevant to both AYA and the clinicians and researchers who have vested interest in their health.[3,9]

In a developmental phase characterized by budding independence and identity formation, access to ICTs can be beneficial,[10] as when AYA of marginalized identities find community online or young users enact adaptive boundary-setting social skills.[11] However, a tension persists between the healthy and developmentally appropriate opportunities ICTs provide and the potential for digitally mediated harm. Historically, discourses around technologically mediated harm have tended to pathologize AYAs use of ICTs. With young people's digital competencies outpacing their caregivers', combined with rapidly evolved post-Web 2.0 privacy norms, AYAs social and sexual lives gained unprecedented reach, a development that was—and remains—alien and disillusioning to many adults.[12] Intrusive monitoring by caregivers, institutions, and clinicians can entrench an adversarial dynamic, as AYA aim to safeguard the spaces in which they exercise independence.[13–15]

The discourses around—and pathologization of—AYAs use of ICTs parallel those of adolescent sexuality, and these paralells prompted the clinicians and researchers of the Adolescent Medicine Trials Network for HIV/AIDS Interventions (ATN) Bioethics Working Group to consider how our lessons learned could be applied to digitally mediated behavioral risk. We have repeatedly encountered the limits of principlist bioethics in application to health services for AYA, legal minors, in particular.[16] Our work exposes the tension between the principles of autonomy and beneficence in delivering interventions to mitigate the risks imposed by pathologized behaviors.

The social norms around adolescent sexuality create barriers to their engagement with providers who could assess sexual health risks and provide appropriate interventions to mitigate them.[17,18] Key among those barriers are concerns about confidentiality, and, relatedly, adolescents' autonomy vis-à-vis consent to care.[19,20] Local statutes dictate the circumstances under which minors may consent to confidential sexual and reproductive health care as well as interventions for other stigmatized health concerns (eg, mental health and substance use disorder).

Legal and ethical frameworks define autonomy and treat it as fact; it exists when one reaches a particular age or social status (eg, marriage)[21] and engages in particular behaviors that conflict with social norms in such a way that their revelation poses risk of harm.[16] However, in our experience, these frameworks often fail to account for the complexities of adolescents' lives. Individual providers and researchers are often left to interpret the space between frameworks designed to address specific and/or discrete circumstances where multiplicitous risks of harm exist. These spaces, in which frameworks fail, create moral conflict for providers and researchers and delay adolescent access to treatment and research. Recent developments in HIV prevention offer a useful example.

In 2012, the Food and Drug Administration (FDA) approved once daily oral tenofovir/emtricitabine (TDF/FTC) for pre-exposure prophylaxis against HIV among adults at risk for sexually acquired infection.[22] However, there were insufficient data on its safety and effectiveness for use with minor adolescents. Thus, ATN scientists developed a protocol to study the safety and tolerability of TDF/FTC among AYA, which called for minor self-consent to enrollment. The requirement for minor self-consent required investigators and institutional review board (IRB) members to grapple with the role of parents in consent processes, a patchwork of local statutes, and the potential social harms of disclosing stigmatized AYA sexualities and/or risk behaviors to caregivers. In later interviews, investigators described experiencing moral conflict due to tension between their scientific and protective duties—conflicts that are examined in depth by Knopf and colleagues.[23] Ultimately, the protocol was approved at only half the sites.[16] In all, it took 6 years for the FDA to approve TDF/FTC for minors, a span of time in which they were denied its prophylactic benefits.

This is one example of circumstances that have given rise to a movement away from discrete definitions of risk, vulnerability, and autonomy and toward an understanding of their intersections and approaches to care that accommodate them.[24,25] Lessons learned in adolescent reproductive and sexual health care can be translated to assessment and mitigation of digitally mediated harms.

The assessment and mitigation of digitally mediated harm must account for the fact that lives of AYA in 2022 are a crosstalk of online and off-line worlds.[26,27] Summative understandings of the effects of ICTs' ubiquity on AYA health and well-being remain largely elusive,[28-30] but the proliferation of affordances they permit is evident.[26] For example, Grindr, Jack'd, and similar "hookup" apps facilitate anonymous location-based sexual encounters with an instantaneity unknown before the smartphone and its geolocational positioning capabilities.[31] ASKfm and Yik Yak offer peer-to-peer features that can be easily reappropriated toward mass anonymous verbal abuse.[32,33] Encountering content that involves sex, illicit drug and alcohol use, and peer-to-peer violence ("fight videos," in particular[34]) has been reported by as many as 84% of Black and/or Hispanic young people.[35] These exposures can drive behavioral risks that transcend, and are accelerated by, both online and off-line and cross-platform interactions: off-line interpersonal conflicts, including physical violence, can be prolonged and catalyzed by online "drama."[34] Digital status-seeking, a form of the impression management encouraged by social media, is linked to increased substance use and sexual risk longitudinally.[36]

However, attempts to generalize dose-response relationships between ICT engagement and behavioral risk often falter[28-30,37] and offer little clinical utility. These phenomena are complex, contextual, and often specific to AYA who inhabit confluences of marginalized identities.[38] For example, coordinated ICT-mediated harassment campaigns have been implicated in the suicides of multiple transgender, nonbinary, and autistic people[39,40]; differential effects by sexual minority status are shown in the associations between cyber-harassment, depressive symptoms, and suicidality among Black AYA[41]; Instagram's own internal user-experience research indicates that pressures to project a "perfect image" on that app fall disproportionately on AYA enduring poverty and, in particular, young women and girls already experiencing mental health-related challenges.[42]

In short, understandings of digitally mediated risk that remain anchored to specific ICTs, or grounded in "normative" or "general" AYA samples, fail to capture the complex interactions between them and the off-line lives of contempory young people, especially those with intersecting marginalized identities. In contrast, a focus on affordances, on *fundamental properties* of the networked ICT environment,[7,8] permits investigators to understand risks that transcend specific platforms and persist across the online and off-line divide. To this end, we engage cross-disciplinary work by boyd.[26] Through long-running ethnographic work with contemporary AYA in the United States, boyd characterized the four inherent affordances of youth digitally networked publics: *persistence* or the durability of online expressions; *searchability*, the ease with which specific digitally networked interactions can be resurfaced, often absent their original context; *spreadability*, the ease with which content can be amplified to mass audiences; and *visibility*, the fundamentally public nature of ICT-enabled sociality. By synthesizing lessons learned across investigational and clinical settings through the lens of these domains, we can develop ethical safeguards to guide the integration of ICT tools into clinical practice with AYA.

Nature of the Problem

Clinicians need a framework for assessing digitally mediated behavioral risk that is rooted in principles and extends beyond platforms. A practice-focused, platform-agnostic digital bioethics is needed, founded on the affordances of digitally networked ICTs, rather than the specific functions of any single technological artifact, although foregrounding autonomy, which, as discussed above, is often contested or restricted in health care and health research contexts.

OBJECTIVE

In this configurative review, we advance behavioral interventions for AYA by mapping a platform-agnostic ethical framework for clinical assessment of digitally mediated behavioral risk. Our framework represents original work conducted by the ATN Bioethics Working Group. The Working Group is composed of clinician-researchers specializing in the assessment of behavioral risk among AYAs, particularly those oppressed along axes of sexuality and gender diversity (often termed "sexual and gender minority" or SGM). Although our focus here is primarily toward the use of ICTs by AYA-serving HIV prevention and treatment providers engaged in behavioral interventions and preventive services,[2,3] we aim to derive insights that can be of use across disciplines.

Approach

To this end, we present initial findings of a systematic literature review, conducted from January 2020 to October 2021, which aimed to synthesize the many *ad hoc* applied ethics that have covered the use of digitally networked ICTs in adolescent HIV prevention. The review's scope adhered to the *methodology, issues, participants* model recommended for systematic reviews of empirical bioethics.[43] The *methodology* focused on longitudinal clinical trials of behavioral interventions or prospective cohort studies; the *issues* focused on ethical principles and applied ethical decision-making guiding the use of ICTs for outreach, case-finding, and recruitment; the *participants* were AYA aged 13 to 29 at risk of HIV acquisition, forward transmission, or viral rebound. Using the subject terms *adolescent HIV, juvenile, teen, young, youth* and full-text terms *attrition, consent, dropout, electronic health record* (EHR), *enrollment, EHRs, network, online, recruitment, retainment, retention,* and *social media*, searches were conducted within EBSCO, Medline, PubMed, PsycInfo, PsycNET, and Proquest. Background, rationale, and full methodological details of the parent review are available as a preregistered narrative protocol at Open Science Framework.[44]

With 6335 retrievals found in initial searches, 1318 duplicates removed, 3928 excluded at title/abstract screening and 946 at full-text review, the analytical sample incudes 12 unique references,[2,45-55] whose key attributes are shown in **Table 1**. These final inclusions describe a range of novel behavioral interventions, implemented within, among, and in partnership with academic medical centers and clinic settings, reliant on ICT platforms. Discrete subsets focused on SGM teens and emerging adults ($n = 3$),[50,51,52] and young men of color ($n = 2$).[54,55] A flow diagram, describing our progression, is shown in **Fig. 1**. Reframing boyd's four affordances of youth networked publics as domains of digitally mediated behavioral risk, we synthesize the lessons learned to date across behavioral HIV prevention interventions, deriving direct practice implications attuned to the developmental benefits of youth networked publics. Finally, informed by the work of Carson and colleagues,[14] and Sussman and DeJong,[15] in adolescent psychiatry, we illustrate these implications through a series of clinical vignettes.

DISCUSSION
Persistence

Social media exist, fundamentally, as for-profit data-harvesting operations, with their interactive features a pretense to elicit behavioral data that is of value to advertisers.[56,57] This reality undergirds concerns expressed in the HIV prevention literature around *persistence*: the durability of records of interactions across networked ICTs.[26] Clicking on a targeted advertisement creates a record of interest, one that may be resurfaced weeks or months later by recommendation algorithms, and targeted ad servers, potentially disclosing stigmatized diagnoses, or oppressed (and closely held) SGM identities,[58] potentially within contexts that may place an AYA user in jeopardy. Relatedly, technological artifacts, such as the "deadnames" that endure in the web addresses of many trans people's Facebook profiles, may expose their assigned sex.[51] For these reasons, HIV behavioral interventions that leverage ICTs have strictly partitioned the social media from the direct interventional aspects of their work[45] and adopted a standard practice of deleting all treatment interactions from chat windows, and clearing browser histories, as a session closes.[50] However, persistence permits asynchronous interaction as well, which can greatly expand access for AYA, who can engage with treatment content, providers, caregivers, and each other, on their own schedules.[46,47]

Searchability

It is through *searchability*, the granulation of online interactions into retrievable terms and sortable categories, which many of the risks inherent in *persistence* are activated: concealable stigmas, instances of harassment and abuse, and illegal acts can achieve discoverability across the life course.[26] Key to the risks inherent in searchability is the stripping of context that occurs when single terms are operationalized as searchable keywords.[45] This loss of nuance may greatly hamper attempts at semi-automated content moderation, which is an important safety protocol for peer-to-peer interventions among AYA.[52] Profanity, which many content moderation platforms flag for removal as a matter of course, may in fact be an important marker of distress,[59] which many AYA prefer to communicate via ICT-mediated spaces.[30] Alternately, terms such as "death note" (the title of a popular anime) may occur in benign contexts. The evolution of youth argot can quickly outpace such systems.[59] However, searchability

Table 1
Attributes of included references

Authors (Year Published)	Intervention	Target Outcome	ICT, Specific Use	Sample Demographics
Bull et al,[45] 2011	*Just/Us*	Impart healthy sexual behaviors, attitudes, and norms	Facebook • Delivery of sexual health education content • Respondent-driven sampling (RDS) recruitment	N = 1,588, aged 16–25 y, U.S. residence
Allison et al,[46] 2012	*n/a*: review of meeting proceedings	—	—	—
Rice et al,[47] 2012	*Have You Heard*	Psychosocial skills building for peer leaders (PLs), participatory creation of digital media encouraging HIV prevention	Facebook MySpace • Community-building • Capturing social network data via "screen grab" • Curation of HIV-prevention content • Amplifying PL reach YouTube • Youth curation of HIV-prevention content	n = 103 "online youth (OY)," recruited via PL networks; no further inclusion criteria applied to OY subsample
Dowshen et al,[48] 2015	*IknowUshould2*	Engage AYA in multimedia campaign and activities encouraging HIV/sexually transmitted infection (STI) testing	iknowushould2.com Facebook Twitter Instagram • Delivery of HIV/STI education content • Locator for HIV/STI testing • Native analytics to track reach, engagement YouTube • Youth sharing STI testing experiences	Primary focus: adolescents 13–17 in Philadelphia. n ≈ 6000 [non-unique] Facebook page visits, n > 1500 unique visits to iknowushould2.com, n = 390 YouTube views

Jones et al.,[49] 2015	Love, Sex, and Choices	Reduce HIV risk through relationship communication, HIV testing, condom use skills	Facebook • Recruitment advertising targeted on urbanity, age, relationship status • Click-through to online screener and consent	N = 40 urban women, aged 18–29 y, in a sexual relationship with ≥1 man in past 3 mo
Lelutiu-Weinbergeret al,[50] 2015	Motivational Interviewing Communication about Health, Attitudes, and Thoughts (MiCHAT)	Reduce condomless anal sex with casual partners, reduce drug use, heavy drinking; increase personal knowledge of sexual risk	Adam4Adam.com • Recruitment via banner ad; Craigslist.com • Recruitment via event promoter; Grindr • Recruitment via pop-up ad; Facebook • Recruitment [unspecified]; • Direct delivery, via anonymous study-specific accounts, of motivational interviewing and cognitive behavioral therapy through chat feature • Recording of session text for clinical supervision	N = 41 young men who have sex with men (YMSM), aged 18–29 y; 46% YMSM of color; 85% gay-identified

(continued on next page)

Table 1
(continued)

Authors (Year Published)	Intervention	Target Outcome	ICT, Specific Use	Sample Demographics
Arayasirikul et al,[51] 2016	*n/a:* longitudinal cohort study	—	Transgenderdate.com Tsdating.com Myredbook.com Craigslist.com Grindr Blendr Scruff OkCupid Tumblr YouTube • Identify young trans-femme study participants Facebook • Identify and retain young trans-femme study participants • Build private group to retain participants longitudinally	*N* = 300 (total RDS + online), assigned male at birth, identified as any gender other than male, aged 16–24 y, San Francisco Bay Area residence
Ybarra et al.,[52] 2016	*Guy2Guy*	Enhance HIV prevention knowledge, motivation, behavioral (eg, condom use) skills; learn healthy relationship skills	Facebook • Recruitment advertising, targeted on location, gender, age, sexual attraction • Click-through to online screener and schedule phone-based consent (including decisional capacity and self-safety assessment) SMS/text messaging • "Text Buddies," pairing anon. participants for discussion, support	*N* = 302, aged 14–18 y, assigned male at birth, identified as male, identified as sexual minority (gay, bisexual, queer), English-literate, exclusive (non-shared) cellphone owners

Matthews et al,[53] 2018	n/a: white paper summarizing workshop series	—	—	—
Patel et al,[54] 2018	Empowering with PrEP (E-PrEP)	Enhance healthcare knowledge, relationship skills; encourage HIV pre-exposure prophylaxis (PrEP) motivation, awareness, and uptake; decrease PrEP stigma	Facebook • Dedicated private groups for each PL, both active/control arms • Exclusive support group for PLs, study staff • Private groups to pretest intervention contents • Targeted advertising to recruit PLs Instagram • Dedicated private feed for each PL, both active/control arms • Targeted advertising to recruit PLs	n = 10 PLs: 18–34 y, Black and/or Latino, male, >500 Facebook or Instagram followers, New York City (NYC) residence n = 152 participants: 18–29 y, Black and/or Latino, male, sexually active, HIV serostatus negative or unknown, NYC residence
Young et al,[55] 2018	n/a: longitudinal cohort study	—	Facebook • Harvesting of Facebook group membership patterns using API • Characterization of group privacy settings	N = 525 [retained at Wave 2], aged 16–29 y, Black/African-American, assigned male at birth, sexually active, South Side Chicago and adjacent metro residence

(continued on next page)

Table 1
(continued)

Authors (Year Published)	Intervention	Target Outcome	ICT, Specific Use	Sample Demographics
Medich et al,[2] 2019	*Using Social Media to Improve Engagement, Retention, and Health Outcomes long the HIV Care Continuum*	HRSA Special Projects of National Significance program, includes 10 demonstration projects at 10 sites	Short message service (SMS)/text messaging WhatsApp, Kik • Outreach, appointment reminders, retention, automated information delivery Facebook Instagram Twitter YouTube • General communication, social support/networking, appointment/care reminders	Expansive range of client/patient populations, AYA newly HIV-seroconverted or out of care/not fully retained in care

Notes: Inclusions are listed chronologically by publication year. As a configurative, interpretive, review, our criteria were inclusive of any applied ethics discussion richer than an IRB approval or regulatory compliance statement. See https://osf.io/4hzqe/ for detailed background, rationale, and methods.[44]

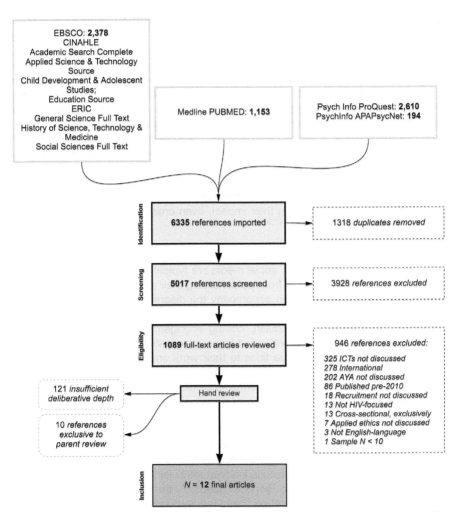

Fig. 1. Flow diagram of progression of systematic literature review. Note: Insufficient deliberative depth = ethical engagements limited to IRB approval or regulatory compliance statements.

demonstrates its greatest promise, and most acute potential dangers, via the instantaneity with which online actors can identify other users by demographic traits—including highly stigmatized SGM identities or medical histories.[51] This can be a boon to case-finding, connecting AYA to services tailored specifically to their needs,[54] or focusing outreach efforts on AYA within zip codes with elevated HIV prevalences.[49] It permits real-time evaluation of such efforts through integrated analytics.[48,49] But given the granularity with which user data are harvested, relinking variables to these traits (in particular geolocational data) can facilitate de-anonymization—a dangerous prospect for many AYA.[46]

Spreadability

Spreadability refers to the rapidity and scale with which information can proliferate across digitally networked ICTs.[26] For earlier generations, sharing a private note passed in class with thousands of strangers with perfect fidelity would be inconceivable; an equivalent act of amplification within the ICT milieu can be close to effortless. This amplification compounds the risks examined above. AYA users often post for an intimate audience of their peers without considering the ramifications of spreadability.[37,59] As such, social media-delivered HIV interventions have taken measures such as eliciting agreements to forgo respective platforms' sharing features[54] or, where possible, disabling them entirely.[54] Such solutions, of course, rely on steadfast consensus among users to remain effective. Agreements can be broken (including by platforms themselves[56]), and screen captures ("screencaps") are a long-established means of circumventing privacy protections and preserving ephemeral (ie, temporary) media.[60] But spreadability grants communicative reach as well, particularly for AYA who lack a voice within traditional media and whose own HIV-prevention messaging is typically treated as more credible by their peers.[55] Youth-curated multimedia can persist, and spread, heightening their impact, even creating opportunities to reconnect with estranged caregivers.[47,54]

Visibility

Pursuant to their business aims, social media are typically "public by default, private by effort,"[26] discouraging users from personalizing their privacy settings by design.[59] The degrees of visibility that can accompany the discrete acts of "liking," "joining," "following," and "sharing" a piece of intervention content, respectively, within Facebook, can be difficult to distinguish, chilling engagement among AYA audiences who may benefit from an intervention but fear stigmatization.[45,55] HIV-prevention staff have, accordingly, applied vague titles to their work and avoided imagery (such as rainbows) that may signal SGM affiliation.[49,53] Even in the absence of searchable traits, hyper-specific media such as gender-transition photos can "out" AYA.[51] Visibility must not imply consent, unilaterally, as norms of privacy may prevail in online settings that are "public" in the purely technical sense.[61] The smartphone lock screen represents another potential vector of visibility: push notifications from outreach staff and providers may be visible to abusive families,[52] particularly in the midst of COVID-related school closures.[62] To mitigate these risks, HIV-prevention staff have scheduled supervisory check-ins to discuss inadvertently visible social media content that may signal unmet psychiatric service needs,[51] formulated stringent "posting etiquette" for use in Facebook groups,[45] and required safety self-assessments for potential participants in peer-to-peer interventions.[52]

Application

Digitally mediated behavioral risk among AYA is complex, platform-agnostic, and highly nuanced. Overlooking this inherent nuance risks pathologizing healthy expressions of ICT-enabled developmental autonomy. As the integration of digital tools into clinical preventive practice continues,[2,3] we reviewed the many *ad hoc* ethical safeguards adopted by HIV researchers as they navigate these tensions, applying the lens of boyd's affordances of youth networked publics.[26] A summary of ICT-mediated risks revealed by our review is shown in **Table 2**.

Finally, we illustrate the application of these risks, and safeguards, respectively, embracing an autonomy-first approach toward fulfilling the often-expressed need among clinicians for contextually adaptive models of digitally mediated behavioral risk.[14,15,64]

Case Vignette 1

Ludmilla is 16, actively exploring agender and trans-feminine identities. She attends a dyadic counseling intervention, applying motivational interviewing (MI) techniques

Table 2
Range of ICT-mediated risks confronted in adolescent HIV prevention practice

Affordance	Risks for AYA
Persistence	Reputational damage linked to user-generated content (UGC) across the life course[47]
	Individual distress linked to UGC recording past experiences, identities, across the life course[51]
	Apathy, forgetfulness, of standards of conduct in longitudinally monitored ICT spaces[45]
	Apathy, forgetfulness, of potential monitoring in longitudinally monitored ICT spaces[51]
	Logging of sensitive interactions on messenger platforms[50]
	Machine-readable keywords exposing sensitive traits to advertisement-targeting algorithms, misc. retention agents[45,49,50]
Searchability	Missed opportunities to intervene on distress, abuse, due to mis-calibrated keywords used by algorithmic content moderation[52,55]
	Missed opportunities to intervene on distress, abuse, due to AYA argot outpacing keyword-based detection[46,51]
	Missed opportunities to intervene on distress, abuse, due to AYA creatively circumnavigating keyword-based content moderation[26]
	Targeting of advertising based on stigmatized traits, affiliations, behaviors[45,49,53]
	Lack of control over amplification, responses, of youth UGC that covers sensitive service/study-related topics[45,46,54]
Spreadability	Unpredictable amplification, context collapse,[63] of UGC intended for peers exclusively[45]
	Unpredictable amplification, context collapse, of UGC intended for service/study staffers exclusively[45,46,48,50,54]
	Ambiguity regarding private vs public nature of UGC in profiles, groups, messages[2,49,51,54,55]
Visibility	Inadvertent disclosure of stigmatized traits via in-group cues in UGC[51]
	Inadvertent exposure of distress, abuse, hate speech to service/study staffer that may trigger crisis response[51]
	Notifications on smartphone lock screens or desktop monitors exposing "closeted" or evolving AYA traits to abusive peers, family[50,52]
	Notifications on smartphone lock screens or desktop monitors exposing stigmatized sexualities to abusive peers, family[50,52]
	Lack of password protection for smartphone access exposing sensitive inbound messages, UGC, service/study interactions[45]

toward Ludmilla's own goal of upholding consistent, assertive, condom use with her multiple concurrent sexual partners.

At session 4, Ludmilla presents euthymic, initially. But she quickly becomes withdrawn. In earlier sessions, she often shared smartphone photos and videos of the people and events she described, swiping expertly through several social media, her smartphone operating system's (OS's) native photo app, and a dating app she favors. Today, she presses the phone flat against her hip, screen down. In response to mild probing, Ludmilla discloses her membership in a private ICT-mediated forum in which she and other trans-feminine members remark on each other's sense of fashion, makeup skills, and respective embodiments of femininity. The group's tone is often good-natured, but can shift abruptly toward targeted, coordinated cruelty. This week, after Ludmilla joined in the mockery of another member, an anonymous account *replied with a brief video, recorded at a recent neighborhood party. In the video, Ludmilla is identifiable, visibly intoxicated, and engaged in a sex act.*

As the forum is tightly restricted, undiscoverable on the open web, and pseudonymous, Ludmilla was at first unconcerned for her broader reputation, despite her humiliation. But on waking this morning, she found that the group member who was the target of her earlier mockery had taken a screencap of Ludmilla's face as it appears in the video, interposed verbally abusive captions, and posted it to a different ICT platform on which Ludmilla connects with her biological family and counseling program resources. Ludmilla is tagged in the post, ensuring that the screencap appears on her profile. Although Ludmilla is able to remove the tag, exercising control over her own profile, several peers in the program have already remarked on the incident in person. Though they are unanimously empathetic and supportive, Ludmilla drops out shortly thereafter.

This vignette illustrates an array of ICT-mediated harms, rooted not in any single platform but their shared affordances. Persistence underlies the acute humiliation and potential reputational damage linked to the screencap once it spread beyond the specific context of the private group, with its more ribald, and possibly ephemeral, norms of conduct.[60] The screencap's visibility among Ludmilla's peers in the program may be a prime contributing factor toward her dropping out of services. It is notable, as well, that the content of the screencap not only violates traditional social mores but also in conflict with her own treatment goals. Such ambivalence toward change is accommodated by MI and many behavioral interventions.[65] But the exposure, in which she was helpless, and the context collapse provoked by the malicious cross-posting,[63] denied her the agency of framing her own decisions and their consequences to her counselor and/or peers.

Private, subcultural, youth networked publics can be spaces of discovery, camaraderie, and social maturation.[11,26] But the group described in Vignette 1 is likely to have driven harm, in equal measure, among its participants. Before her own victimization, Ludimilla was, evidently, a perpetrator of abuse of other group participants. As Carson and colleagues note, acknowledging the possibility of perpetration, alongside victimization, is essential to assessing for AYA digital safety.[14] As well, although a program-wide code of conduct may have discouraged AYA service users from interacting outside of the interventions context,[45,49] direct AYA-empowering digital safety self-assessment and skills-building would likely be the most effective safeguard against the risks illustrated in Vignette 1.[52,66,67] Still, these safeguards rely, predominantly, on mutually reciprocated trust among young users.[54,58] This can be a difficult equilibrium to maintain, but one that may be bolstered by cultivating injunctive norms against cross-platform violations of trust,[68] and embracing rhetorics of community safety and digital citizenship among AYA.[69]

Case Vignette 2

Luisa is a community health worker, facilitating an outpatient group intervention for young adults who aim to reduce their drug use. Justin, 19, is among the group's most dedicated members. After a daylong blackout and a bout of protracted, dissociative anxiety, Justin's goal is to reduce his use of alcohol and MDMA [3,4-methylenedioxymethamphetamine, aka "Ecstasy" or "Molly"[70]], particularly in combination. Justin resides, sporadically, with his stepfather. Justin has struggled to find regular employment. His housing options, in turn, are scant. Justin fears his stepfather, who is unaware of the extent of Justin's substance use, and has threatened to call law enforcement if he suspects the use of drugs on his property.

Justin suspects his stepfather has attempted to access his password-protected smartphone and knows with certainty his stepfather monitors his only identifiable social media account. Luísa is aware of this because her clinic conducts a digital safety assessment at intake. The digital safety assessment was developed after several members complained that the group's use of social media for contact led to aggressive for-profit recovery center ads "following them" around the web. Justin's digital safety assessment indicated a need for a protocol for Luísa to safely contact him. Luísa uses an encrypted messenger app to contact Justin during the daily window in which she knows he is outside of the home. As an added safeguard, Luísa and Justin customized the app's settings and those of the smartphone's native OS to ensure service-related notifications do not appear on Justin's lock screen.

Luísa, concerned about Justin's safety, contacts him per protocol. After 45 minutes, well in excess of his average response time, Justin has not replied. Once, a month earlier, Justin relapsed, losing his phone and replacing it with a different model with an unfamiliar OS, which necessitated careful reworking of his and Luísa's outreach protocols. After another hour, Luísa considers breaking protocol by checking Justin's "unfiltered" pseudonymous social media account or chancing a text message outside of their established window for safe outreach.

In this vignette, a range of safeguards described by this review have been integrated into Justin's and Luísa's routine clinical encounters. This integration would have been impossible if not for the insights yielded by the digital safety self-assessment at intake,[52] which ensured that a firmly mandated client-centered protocol was in place to protect Justin from his stepfather's surveillance. Of note, the consequences of this surveillance exist despite Justin's having attained the legal age of majority.

But the juncture at which Vignette 2 closes does not invite easy resolution. Justin may be in physical or medical danger, and his true social media may offer clarity on his circumstances. Although Justin's social media are visible, they are not searchable by anybody who does not know his private handle. His expectations concerning their privacy, regardless of their default visibility, remain unclear. Ultimately, Justin is an adult, and his expectations around digital safety have been documented. Falling back on the mandates of the protocol, despite their now-evident gaps, would be the course of action that most closely aligns with respect for his (legally enshrined, if still practically constrained) personal autonomy.

SUMMARY

As clinical encounters increasingly rely on the same digitally networked ICTs that can drive behavioral risk among AYA, it is imperative that clinicians embrace concrete ethical safeguards to guide their adoption of these same digital tools. By moving our understandings beyond reductive frameworks and toward adaptive, cross-disciplinary understandings of today's rich digital AYA milieu, we can integrate robust safeguards into current practice and future behavioral interventions. As an initial step to this end, we reviewed *ad hoc* digital ethical safeguards adopted by adolescent HIV prevention researchers and practitioners, configuring them through the lens of boyd's four affordances of youth networked publics. Integrating these safeguards into clinical practice, while upholding patient/client autonomy, will represent important strides toward empowering young people to protect themselves from the potential harms examined here.

CLINICS CARE POINTS

- Clinicians must build digital safety knowledge and skills responsive to the unique needs of respective adolescents and young adults (AYA) subpopulations.[66,67]

- Clinicians should integrate digital safety assessments (including *self*-assessments) into intake and routine clinical encounters with AYA.
- Clinicians and their practices should avoid service/study branding that signals affiliation with stigmatized traits.
- Clinicians should enact routine re-consenting and digital privacy refreshers for service/study-enrolled AYA who engage in interactive communication technology (ICT)-mediated contacts.
- Clinicians should maintain awareness of platform functionality updates that may drastically alter an ICT's key affordances.

ACKNOWLEDGMENTS

This work was supported by the Eunice Kennedy Shriver National Institute of Child Health and Human Development, Adolescent Medicine Trials Network for HIV/AIDS Interventions (ATN) as part of the Scale It Up Program (U19HD089875; PI: Naar). S.J. Skeen is supported in part by a Garvin Shands Saunders Foundation scholarship. We are grateful to Celina Meyer for assistance in screening titles and abstracts, and to Sylvie Naar for convening the ATN Bioethics Working Group.

DISCLOSURE

S.J. Skeen is a paid advisor to Waverider, which builds customizable DBT-CBT eHealth tools. S.K. Shaw Green declares no conflicts of interests. A.S. Knopf declares no conflicts of interests.

REFERENCES

1. Pew Research Center. Teens. Social Media & Technology; 2018. Available at: https://www.pewresearch.org/internet/2018/05/31/teens-social-media-technology-2018/. Accessed December 10, 2021.
2. Medich M, Swendeman DT, Comulada WS, et al. Promising approaches for engaging youth and young adults living with HIV in HIV primary care using social media and mobile technology interventions: protocol for the SPNS social media initiative. JMIR Res Protoc 2019;8(1):e10681.
3. Wong CA, Madanay F, Ozer EM, et al. Digital health technology to enhance adolescent and young adult clinical preventive services: affordances and challenges. J Adolesc Health 2020;67:S24–33.
4. National Institutes of Health (NIH). NIH RePORTER. Available at: https://reporter.nih.gov/. Accessed November 15, 2021.
5. Naar S, Parsons JT, Stanton BF. Adolescent Trials Network for HIV-AIDS Scale It Up program: protocol for a rational and overview. JMIR Res Protoc 2019;8(2):e11204.
6. Hightow-Weidman LB, Muessig K, Rosenberg E, et al. University of North Carolina/Emory Center for Innovative Technology (iTech) for addressing the HIV epidemic among adolescents and young adults in the United States: protocol and rationale for center development. JMIR Res Protoc 2018;7(8):e10365.
7. Norman D. The psychology of everyday things. New York: Basic Books; 1988.
8. Gaver WW. Technology affordances. CHI '91: Proceedings of the SIGCHI Conference on Human Factors in Computing Systems. 1991; 27–2. New Orleans, LA. doi:0-89791-383-3/91/0004/0079.
9. Moreno MA, Uhls YT. Applying an affordances approach and a developmental lens to approach adolescent social media use. Digit Health 2019. https://doi.org/10.1177/2055207619826678. Epub ahead of print.

10. Montgomery KC, Chester J, Milosevic T. Children's privacy in the big data era: research opportunities. Pediatrics 2017;140(S2):e20161758.

11. Rafalow MH. N00bs, trolls, and idols: boundary-making among digital youth. In: Blais SL, Claster PN, Claster SM, editors. Technology and youth: growing up in a digital world. Bingley, UK: Emerald Books; 2015. p. 243–66.

12. Marwick A. To catch a predator? The MySpace moral panic. First Monday 2008; 13(6). Available at: https://firstmonday.org/article/view/2152/1966.

13. Marwick A, Fontaine C, boyd d. Nobody sees it, nobody gets mad": social media, privacy, and personal responsibility among low-SES youth. Soc Med Soc 2017; 3(2):1–14.

14. Carson NJ, Gansner M, Khang J. Assessment of digital media use in the adolescent psychiatric evaluation. Child Adolesc Psychiatr Clin N Am 2018;27:133–43.

15. Sussman N, DeJong SM. Ethical considerations for mental health clinicians working with adolescents in the digital age. Curr Psychiatry Rep 2018;20:113.

16. Gilbert AL, Knopf AS, Fortenberry JD, et al. Adolescent self-consent for biomedical HIV prevention research. J Adolesc Health 2015;57(1):113–9.

17. Santelli JS, Kantor LM, Grilo SA, et al. Abstinence-only-until-marriage: an updated review of U.S. policies and programs and their impact. J Adolesc Health 2017;61(3):P273–80.

18. American Public Health Association. Abstinence and U.S. Abstinence Only Education Policies: Ethical and Human Rights Concerns. Policy Number: 200610. 2006. Available at: https://www.apha.org/policies-and-advocacy/public-health-policy-statements/policy-database/2014/07/18/14/05/abstinence-and-us-abstinence-only-education-policies-ethical-and-human-rights-concerns. Accessed December 22, 2021.

19. Ford C, English A, Sigman G, et al. Confidential health care for adolescents: position paper of the Society for Adolescent Medicine. J Adolesc Health 2004;35(3): P160–7.

20. Brittain AW, Brieno ACL, Pazol K, et al. Youth-friendly family planning services for young people: a systematic review update. Am J Prev Med 2018;55(5):725–35.

21. Centers for Disease Control and Prevention. State Laws that Enable a Minor to Provide Informed Consent to Receive HIV and STD Services. 2021. Available at: https://www.cdc.gov/hiv/policies/law/states/minors.html. Accessed December 22, 2021.

22. Centers for Disease Control and Prevention. CDC statement on FDA approval of drug for HIV prevention 2012. Available at: https://www.cdc.gov/nchhstp/newsroom/2012/fda-approvesdrugstatement.html. Accessed March 15, 2022.

23. Knopf AS, Gilbert AL, Zimet GD, et al. The Adolescent Medicine Trials Network for HIV/AIDS Interventions. Moral conflict and competing duties in the initiation of a biomedical HIV prevention trial with minor adolescents. AJOB Empir Bioeth 2017; 8(3):145–52.

24. McGregor KA, Hensel DJ, Waltz AC, et al. Adolescent sexual behavior: perspectives of investigators, IRB members, and IRB staff about risk categorization and IRB approval. IRB Ethics Hum Res 2017;39(4):17–20.

25. Ott MA. Vulnerability in HIV prevention research with adolescents, reconsidered. J Adolesc Health 2014;54:629–30.

26. boyd d. It's complicated: the social lives of networked teens. New Haven, CT: Yale University Press; 2014.

27. Saleh F, Grudzinkas A, Judge A, editors. Adolescent sexual behavior in the digital age: considerations for clinicians, legal professionals and educators. New York: Oxford University Press; 2014.

28. Twenge JM, Joiner TE, Rogers ML, et al. Increases in depressive symptoms, suicide-related outcomes, and suicide rates among U.S. adolescents after 2010 and links to increased new media screen time. Clin Psychol Sci 2018; 6(1):3–17.

29. Vuorre M, Orben A, Przybylski AK. There is no evidence that associations between adolescents' digital technology engagement and mental health problems have increased. Clin Psychol Sci 2021;9(5):823–35.

30. Marchant A, Hawton K, Stewart A, et al. A systematic review of the relationship between internet use, self-harm and suicidal behaviour in young people: the good, the bad and the unknown. PLoS ONE 2017;12(8):e0181722.

31. Van De Wiele C, Tom Tong S. Breaking boundaries: the uses & gratifications of Grindr. UbiComp '14: International Joint Conference on Ubiquitous and Pervasive Computing. September 2014;13–17. Seattle, WA. https://doi.org/10.1145/2632048.2636070.

32. Ashktorab Z, Haber E, Golbeck J, et al. Beyond cyberbullying: self-disclosure, harm and social support on ASKfm. WebSci '17: 9th International ACM Web Science Conference. 2017;26–28. Troy, NY. https://doi.org/10.1145/3091478.3091499.

33. Black EW, Mezzina K, Thompson LA. Anonymous social media – understanding the content and context of Yik Yak. Comput Human Behav 2016;57:17–22.

34. Stevens R, Gilliard-Matthews S, Dunaev J, et al. The digital hood: social media use among youth in disadvantaged neighborhoods. New Media Soc 2017; 19(6):950–67.

35. Stevens R, Bleakley A, Hennessy M, et al. #digital hood: engagement with risk content on social media among Black and Hispanic youth. J Urban Health 2019;96:74–82.

36. Nesi J, Prinstein MJ. In search of likes: longitudinal associations between adolescents' digital status seeking and health risk behaviors. J Clin Child Adolesc Psychol 2019;48(5):740–8.

37. James C, Davis K, Charmaraman L, et al. Digital life and youth well-being, social connectedness, empathy, and narcissism. Pediatrics 2017;140(S2):e20161758.

38. Bailey J, Burkell J. Tech-facilitated violence: thinking structurally and intersectionally. J Gend Based Viol 2021;5(3):531–42.

39. Wodinsky S. The worst site on the web gets DDoS'd after being connected to prominent developer's suicide. Gizmodo 2021. Available at: https://gizmodo.com/the-worst-site-on-the-web-gets-ddosd-after-being-connec-1847196197. Accessed December 5, 2021.

40. Vu AV, Wilson L, Chua YT, et al. ExtremeBB: enabling large-scale research into extremism, the manosphere and their correlation by online forum data. arXiv 2021. Available at: https://arxiv.org/pdf/2111.04479.pdf.

41. Mereish EH, Sheskier M, Hawthorne D, et al. Sexual orientation disparities in mental health and substance use among Black American young people in the U.S.A.: effects of cyber and bias-based victimization. Cult Health Sex 2019; 21(9):985–98.

42. Instagram. Teen mental health deep dive. 2021. Available at: https://about.fb.com/news/2021/09/research-teen-well-being-and-instagram/. Accessed December 5, 2021.

43. Strech D, Synofzik M, Marckmann G. Systematic reviews of empirical bioethics. J Med Ethics 2008;34:472–7.

44. Shaw Green SK, Skeen SJ. Mapping the digital bioethics embraced by adolescent HIV prevention researchers recruiting online: protocol for a systematic

literature review and critical interpretive synthesis. Open Science Framework 2021. Available at: https://osf.io/4hzqe/.

45. Bull SS, Breslin LT, Wright EE, et al. Case study: an ethics case study of HIV prevention research on Facebook: The Just/Us study. J Pediatr Psychol 2011;36: 1082–92.

46. Allison S, Bauermeister JA, Bull S, et al. The intersection of youth, technology, and new media with sexual health: moving the research agenda forward. J Adolesc Health 2012;51:207–12.

47. Rice E, Tulbert E, Cederbaum J, et al. Mobilizing homeless youth for HIV prevention: a social network analysis of the acceptability of a face-to-face and online social networking intervention. Health Educ Res 2012;27:226–36.

48. Dowshen N, Lee S, Lehman M, et al. IknowUshould2: feasibility of a youth-driven social media campaign to promote STI and HIV testing among adolescents in Philadelphia. AIDS Behav 2015;19:S106–11.

49. Jones R, Lacroix LJ, Nolte K. Is your man stepping out?" An online pilot study to evaluate acceptability of a guide-enhanced HIV prevention soap opera video series and feasibility of recruitment by Facebook advertising. J Assoc Nurses AIDS Care 2015;26:368–86.

50. Lelutiu-Weinberger C, Pachankis JE, Gamarel KE, et al. Feasibility, acceptability, and preliminary efficacy of a live-chat social media intervention to reduce HIV risk among young men who have sex with men. AIDS Behav 2015;19:1214–27.

51. Arayasirikul S, Chen Y-H, Jin H, et al. A Web 2.0 and epidemiology mash-up: using respondent-driven sampling in combination with social network site recruitment to reach young transwomen. AIDS Behav 2016;20:1265–74.

52. Ybarra ML, Prescott TL, Phillips GL, et al. Ethical considerations in recruiting online and implementing a text messaging-based HIV prevention program with gay, bisexual, and queer adolescent males. J Adolesc Health 2016;59:44–9.

53. Matthews AK, Rak K, Anderson E, et al. White paper from a CTSA workshop series on special and underserved populations: enhancing investigator readiness to conduct research involving LGBT populations. J Clin Transl Sci 2018;2: 193–200.

54. Patel VV, Ginsburg Z, Golub SA, et al. Empowering with PrEP (E-PrEP), a peer-led social media–based intervention to facilitate HIV preexposure prophylaxis adoption among young Black and Latinx gay and bisexual men: protocol for a cluster randomized controlled trial. JMIR Res Protoc 2008;7:e11375.

55. Young LE, Fujimoto K, Schneider JA. HIV prevention and sex behaviors as organizing mechanisms in a Facebook group affiliation network among young Black men who have sex with men. AIDS Behav 2018;22:3324–34.

56. Montgomery KC. Youth and surveillance in the Facebook era: policy interventions and social implications. Telecommun Policy 2015;39:771–86.

57. Amnesty International. Surveillance Giants: How the Business Model of Google and Facebook Threatens Human Rights. 2019. Available at: https://www.amnesty.org/en/documents/pol30/1404/2019/en/. Accessed December 22, 2021.

58. Bender JL, Cyr AB, Arbuckle L, et al. Ethics and privacy implications of using the internet and social media to recruit participants for health research: a privacy-by-design framework for online recruitment. J Med Internet Res 2017;19(4):e104.

59. Perez Vallejos E, Koene A, Carter CJ, et al. Accessing online data for youth mental health research: meeting the ethical challenges. Philos Technol 2019; 32:87–110.

60. Charteris J, Gregory S, Masters Y. 'Snapchat', youth subjectivities and sexuality: disappearing media and the discourse of youth innocence. Gend Educ 2018; 30(2):205–21.

61. Franzke AS, Bechmann A, Zimmer M, et al. Association of Internet Researchers. Internet Res Ethical Guidel 3.0. 2019. Available at: https://aoir.org/reports/ethics3.pdf. Accessed December 22, 2021.

62. Pfefferbaum B. Challenges for child mental health raised by school closure and home confinement during the COVID-19 pandemic. Curr Psychiatry Rep 2021; 23:65.

63. Marwick AE, boyd d. I tweet honestly, I tweet passionately: Twitter users, context collapse, and the imagined audience. New Media Soc 2010;13(1):114–33.

64. Alessi NE, Alessi VA. New media and an ethics analysis model for child and adolescent psychiatry. Child Adolesc Psychiatr Clin N Am 2008;17:67–92.

65. Koken J, Outlaw A, Green-Jones M. Sexual risk reduction. In: Naar-King S, Suarez M, editors. Motivational interviewing with adolescents and young adults. New York: The Guilford Press; 2011. p. 106–11.

66. Electronic Frontier Foundation. Surveill Self-Defense: LGBTQ Youth. Available at: https://ssd.eff.org/en/playlist/lgbtq-youth. Accessed December 22, 2021.

67. Grindr for Equality. Grindr Holistic Security Guide. Available at: https://www.grindr.com/g4e/G4E-HolisticSecurityGuide-English.pdf. Accessed December 22, 2021.

68. Dym B, Fiesler C. Social norm vulnerability and its consequences for privacy and safety in an online community. Proc ACM Human-Computer Interaction 2020; 155:1–24.

69. Jones LM, Mitchell KJ. Defining and measuring youth digital citizenship. New Media Soc 2016;18(9):2063–79.

70. National Institute on Drug Abuse. MDMA (Ecstasy) Abuse Research Report. 2017. Available at: https://nida.nih.gov/publications/research-reports/mdma-ecstasy-abuse/Introduction. Accessed March 12, 2022.

Self-Management Frameworks for Youth Living with Human Immunodeficiency Virus

Karen Kolmodin MacDonell, PhD[a],*, Sylvie Naar, PhD[b]

KEYWORDS

- Adolescents and emerging adults • Self-management • HIV treatment cascade
- Chronic disease management • Behavioral interventions

KEY POINTS

- Adolescents and emerging adults continue to represent a substantial proportion of new HIV diagnoses.
- HIV self-management is critical and complex, particularly during adolescence and emerging adulthood.
- Youth can now lead essentially healthy lives with currently available HIV medical care regimens, but there are many challenges to effectively managing HIV.
- For youth living with HIV, self-management goes beyond activities specifically related to treating and caring for HIV along the treatment cascade and includes managing substance use and sexual health because of the impact these activities have on HIV transmission and disease progression.

SELF-MANAGEMENT FRAMEWORKS FOR YOUTH LIVING WITH HUMAN IMMUNODEFICIENCY VIRUS

Great progress has been made over the past 30 years in the prevention and treatment of HIV. Combination antiretroviral treatment (ART) has transformed infection with HIV from a rapidly debilitating, fatal disease into a chronic condition with high potential for a healthy life for multiple decades.[1,2] Combined with widely available, accurate and rapid HIV-testing, preexposure prophylaxis (PrEP) for individuals

---

[a] Wayne State University School of Medicine, Family Medicine and Public Health Sciences, IBio 6135 Woodward Avenue, Behavioral Health, H206, Detroit, MI 48202, USA; [b] Florida State University, Center for Translational Behavioral Science, 2010 Levy Avenue Building B, Suite B0266, Tallahassee, FL 32310, USA
* Corresponding author.
E-mail address: karen.macdonell@wayne.edu

Pediatr Clin N Am 69 (2022) 759–777
https://doi.org/10.1016/j.pcl.2022.04.007
0031-3955/22/© 2022 Elsevier Inc. All rights reserved.

at high-risk, and universal viral suppression for those infected, an AIDS-free generation and the end to the global AIDS epidemic are ambitious, but achievable national and global goals.[3,4] Despite growing optimism about this potentially achievable outcome, the epidemic remains a major cause of morbidity and mortality worldwide, particularly among adolescents and emerging/young adults (hereafter called "youth") and disproportionately among sexual, gender, and/or racial and ethnic minority youth.[5] Between 2014 and 2018, new HIV diagnoses actually decreased 15% among youth (ages 13–24) overall. Despite this, in 2018, 21% of all new HIV diagnoses in the United States and dependent areas were among youth ages 13 to 24, with gay and bisexual young men disproportionately represented in new diagnoses.[6]

Managing Human Immunodeficiency Virus Among Youth

Adolescents and emerging adults represent a substantial proportion of new HIV diagnoses, but nearly half of all youth living with HIV in the US are not aware that they are infected.[6] Even among those who are aware of their HIV-positive status, far too many struggle with managing HIV as many do not seek treatment, do not remain in treatment over time, fail to take ART as prescribed, particularly over the long-term, and are ultimately not able to achieve HIV viral suppression.[6] Viral suppression occurs when ART reduces a person's HIV in the blood to an undetectable level, and is essential to maintaining the health of the infected person and preventing further transmission of the virus to other people.[7] The Centers for Disease Control and Prevention (CDC) estimate that only 63.3% of adolescents and emerging adults ages 13 to 24 years with diagnosed HIV infection have achieved viral suppression (in this case, as defined by viral load <200 copies/mL of blood).[8] In 2018, for every 100 young people living with HIV in the US, 55 knew their HIV status, 79 received some HIV medical care, 58 were retained in care, and 60 were virally suppressed.[6] In a recent study of 1411 young people living with HIV ages 12 to 24 across the US, 75% were linked to HIV medical care at adolescent HIV care sites, 59% were engaged in care, and 34% were retained in care. However, only 34% had started ART and 12% had attained viral suppression.[9] These findings strongly suggest that even after youth are linked to an HIV medical care program, a low proportion demonstrate successful disease management including taking ART to achieve viral suppression and attending HIV clinical health care appointments.

The CDC has noted numerous challenges that may make it particularly difficult for adolescents and emerging adults to access the tools they need to manage HIV.[6] Complex, multilevel factors beyond just individual-level factors may contribute to disparities in HIV rates, morbidity, and mortality, particularly in sexual, gender, and/or racial minority youth.[10] Within US samples, barriers may include social and economic challenges such as low income, recent homelessness, recent incarceration, and/or lack of or unstable health insurance.[6] These barriers may be even more significant in minoritized communities because of various forms of discrimination such as homophobia and transphobia. Discrimination may result in a lack of culturally responsive health care,[11] and unequal and unfair treatment across social systems such as housing, education, and criminal justice.[10,12] To end the HIV epidemic, we must find better ways to reduce the risk of HIV transmission, link youth to HIV health care, improve adherence to the HIV care regimen, and keep youth retained in care and adherent to medication over time with the goal of viral suppression. Moreover, we must continue to recognize that sexual, gender, and/or racial/minority youth face significant disparities in all steps of HIV prevention and treatment and beyond.

Managing Substance Use and Sexual Risk Among Youth Living with Human Immunodeficiency Virus

Substance use, particularly marijuana, tobacco, and alcohol use, has been found to be common among youth living with HIV,[13–17] with higher substance use associated with unsuppressed viral load in US and global samples of people living with HIV.[18] Nearly 25% percent of youth living with HIV reported weekly or greater alcohol use in a large multi-site study of youth in clinical care across the United States.[19] Moreover, in this study, nearly 33% of youth reported weekly or more frequent tobacco use, 27.5% reported marijuana use, and 22.5% reported other illicit drug use. Young men-who-have-sex-with-men were more likely to report each substance use behavior, while transgender women were more likely to report marijuana and other illicit drug use than youth in other demographic categories. Overall, youth living with HIV who were involved in the criminal justice system had unstable housing, engaged in condomless (risky) sex, and/or did not take ART as prescribed by their HIV care physician were more likely to use substances in this study.

Substance use may have multiple detrimental social, psychological, and health consequences for youth living with HIV.[19] Alcohol use, in particular, has been found to have synergistic and additive effects on health and common HIV-related comorbidities.[20] Studies with adults living with HIV demonstrate a relationship between alcohol use and accelerated HIV disease,[18,21,22] and there is increasing concern about the detrimental effects of HIV and alcohol use on brain functioning.[23] Alcohol use has also been linked to increased risk behaviors for HIV transmission,[24] poor adherence to ART,[25] worsening disease progression,[26] and has been found to impact HIV care and outcomes at every level (HIV testing, diagnosis, connection to HIV health care, HIV treatment, and viral suppression).[20]

Within adolescents and emerging adults, we know that risk behaviors tend to cluster, with substance use behaviors often cooccurring with other risk behaviors[22] and linked to increased sexual risk behaviors in samples of youth in the US.[18,27,28] Alcohol use, in particular, has been associated with increased risk of engaging in unprotected sex.[24,29] Higher prevalence of sexually transmitted infections (STIs) has also been linked to substance use frequency and/or problematic level of substance use among youth living with HIV in clinical care settings, particularly alcohol, marijuana, and other drugs.[30] Overall, navigating their developing roles as sexual beings is complex for all youth, but even more so for youth with chronic diseases impacting sexual activity or youth whose sexual orientation may increase their likelihood of sexual activity with HIV + individuals.[31] Among adolescent sexual minority males (ages 14–19), one of the groups of youth at elevated risk for HIV transmission in the United States, a recent meta-analysis found that an estimated 67% recently had sex. Among these youth, 44% had condomless anal intercourse within the past 6 months, 50% did not use a condom at last sex, and 32% used alcohol or drugs during their last sexual experience.[32] Despite these increased risks in adolescents and emerging adults, particularly sexual minority youth, there is insufficient research focused on their unique HIV risk and prevention needs; moreover, research evaluating sexual risk-taking, and even more so emerging sexual health needs, among youth living with HIV is limited.

Self-Management of Human Immunodeficiency Virus as a Multi-Faceted Chronic Condition

Despite the multiple challenges facing youth living with HIV, they can now lead essentially healthy lives with currently available HIV medical care regimens. To achieve this goal, a youth must determine their HIV status and become committed to the managing points along the HIV treatment cascade. The "HIV treatment cascade," sometimes referred to as the "HIV care continuum," is a model of the steps people living with HIV go through from initial diagnosis of HIV to achieving viral suppression (**Fig. 1**). Once HIV-positive status is confirmed, the youth must immediately engage with the HIV care system, initiate ART, and comprehend and embrace the necessity of proper medication adherence, be retained in HIV care, and, finally, maintain viral suppression. Collectively, these steps along the HIV treatment cascade are also what has been called, *HIV self-management,* defined as "strategies to help individuals ...and their caregivers better understand and manage their illness and [/or] improve their health behaviors."[33] This is critical for youth living with HIV because higher self-management has been linked to better adherence to ART, successful viral suppression, and more consistent condom use.[34]

For youth living with HIV, self-management goes beyond activities specifically related to treating and caring for HIV along the treatment cascade (eg, taking ART, attending clinic appointments) and includes managing substance use and sexual health because of the impact these activities have on HIV transmission and disease progression.[17,25,26] HIV self-management is critical and complex at any age, but may be especially challenging among adolescents and emerging adults as they transition from a largely dependent to a more independent status ("transition to self-management")[35] during developmental periods marked by: identity exploration and self-focus; development of new social networks, increased opportunities and choices, both positive and risk-laden; increased independence and risk-taking behavior (demonstrating the highest level of risk behavior engagement among all age groups); and, decreased parental support and oversight.[36-40] Unfortunately, many youth living with HIV have poor HIV self-management behaviors, including medication adherence[41,42] and retention in HIV care[43] compared with other age groups. Additionally, the prevalence of most kinds of substance use and abuse, including alcohol use,[14,19,44,45] is highest during the transition to adulthood.[38]

A significant substance use concern is smoking behaviors that are highly prevalent among youth living with HIV.[46] Smoking is especially concerning given the increased risk for cardiovascular disease associated with HIV.[47] Using electronic health records, our group has shown that higher cardiovascular disease risk is associated with elevated viral load and reduced immune function.[48] Thus, in addition to reducing smoking, self-management behaviors include general health behaviors that prevent cardiovascular diseases such as nutrition and physical activity, as well as preventive vaccines such as HPV and COVID-19. Additionally, youth living with HIV have to manage side effects resulting from ART medications,[49] as well as potential drug–drug interactions if they are prescribed a medication for any chronic condition beyond HIV (eg, cardiovascular or analgesic medication).[50] As with other chronic conditions, effective self-management is an essential aspect of managing disease, with particular focus on illness prevention and wellness promotion.[51]

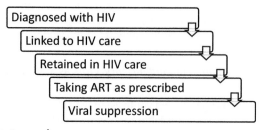

Fig. 1. HIV treatment cascade.

Theoretic Foundation of the Concept of Self-Management

The broad concept of self-management emerged simultaneously within the substance abuse and chronic health condition literatures, and has particular relevance for youth living with HIV given the developmental tasks and challenges of adolescence and emerging adulthood. These challenges include increasing independence, shifting social and emotional supports, transition from pediatric to adult care, increased risk-taking behaviors, and so forth, as described above. For youth living with HIV who are also members of minoritized communities (eg, sexual, gender, and/or racial or ethnic minority groups), these challenges may be compounded with additional exploration of identity, fear of disclosure and/or stigma, and experienced or anticipated stigma.[52]

Self-Management of Substance Use

In substance abuse research, approaches to prevention and intervention in young people have shifted from social influences promoting substance use[53] to cognitive-behavioral personal and social skills needed to resist substance use.[54] Current research now identifies individual-level *self-management skills* such as self-control, decision-making, self-reinforcement, and problem solving as core competencies that protect against substance use and abuse.[55,56] Self-management skills are closely tied to increasing autonomy and agency that characterize the transition to adulthood. These skills are not usually fully developed until adulthood, and mature at different rates across individuals.[56] There is consistent evidence from cross-sectional research that higher self-management skills, particularly planfulness, problem solving, self-reinforcement, and cognitive effort, are linked to lower levels of substance use.[57] Higher self-management skills in early adolescence may even be protective of substance use later in adolescence and early adulthood.[56] There is also evidence that the underlying development of self-management skills is linked to neurologic maturation and connectivity between areas of the brain responsible for self-control and decision-making.[58] Neurobiological research has found regions of the brain responsible for self-management skills do not reach maturity until late adolescence or early adulthood, while those brain areas associated with the processing of social and emotional stimuli develop much earlier in early adolescence.[58] This is one explanation for youths' susceptibly to risk-taking behaviors, including substance use, particularly in the presence of peers.[59]

Self-Management of Pediatric Chronic Medical Conditions

The increased prevalence of chronic health conditions combined with significant reductions in mortality rates for many pediatric conditions has changed how we view chronic health conditions during adolescence and into emerging adulthood.[60] More emphasis has shifted to managing chronic health conditions over the long-term, from childhood, through adolescence, and into the transition to adulthood. In the pediatric chronic health condition literature, *self-management* emerged as a term to broaden the focus from treatment compliance,[61] to medication adherence, and finally, to the range of skills necessary to independently manage a chronic medical condition.[62] Self-management of chronic health conditions refers to the ability to manage symptoms, treatments, lifestyle changes, and consequences of health conditions,[63] take responsibility for one's own health, and use resources effectively toward living a healthier life. This requires skills around problem-solving, goal-setting, and action-planning,[64] as well as specific health behaviors required to effectively manage illness (eg, medication adherence, appointment-keeping).

Self-management may be a particularly useful conceptual framework for adolescents and emerging adults with chronic health conditions, as it assumes autonomy and increasing responsibility for one's own health decisions during the transition from childhood to adulthood. Most chronically ill youth and their caregivers coordinate much of their health care themselves; moreover, many chronic care models that have been incorporated into health care services and clinics do not address the specific needs of youth, particularly as they transition to increasingly independent care.[65] Adolescents and emerging adults face various physical, emotional, and social changes that are often particularly challenging for youth living with chronic health conditions and may negatively impact illness self-management. However, research on youth with chronic conditions has also identified multiple factors that may facilitate better self-management behaviors, including psychosocial factors (eg, higher self-efficacy,[66] positive attitude toward illness,[67] perception of self as "normal" compared with peers[68]), knowledge about their illness, more effective coping skills, and sharing self-management tasks with parents during the transition to independence.[69]

Adapting Frameworks for the Self-Management of Human Immunodeficiency Virus in Youth

Self-management of HIV, and relatedly substance use and sexual health, during adolescence and emerging adulthood is often complicated by the physical, cognitive, and social changes that occur during the process of adolescent development and the challenges associated with both adolescence and emerging adulthood. The concept of self-management emerged from various literatures, most notably substance use and chronic health condition management. A guiding self-management framework may be useful to understand how components of self-management interact and combine to influence HIV-related health behavior and HIV clinical outcomes. Several frameworks have been proposed to illustrate the self-management of HIV in adolescents and emerging adults. These frameworks emphasize different barriers and facilitators to self-management, with varying strengths and weaknesses based on their approaches to understanding HIV self-management.

Five components model

The Five Components Model (**Fig. 2**) was derived from the National Institute of Nursing Research's workshop on improving the quality of life for individuals with chronic health conditions.[33] In this model, self-management is viewed as multiple strategies to help people with chronic conditions and their caregivers better understand and manage their illness and improve their health behaviors. Thus, this model includes the consideration of factors, largely individual-level, that may hinder or facilitate effective illness self-management. Naar, Parsons, and Stanton[70] adapted this model for youth living with HIV, proposing 5 essential skills around illness self-management. These essential skills include: problem solving, decision making, resource utilization, forming of a patient/health care provider partnership, and taking action.[51,71] Problem solving involves understanding the problems, options, as well as downsides and advantages of each option or behavior. This is linked to both decision-making or the youth deciding what works best for themselves, and resource utilization, or the logistical and financial factors that may impact the initial decision. The provider relationship is linked to all steps within this model, and all components have reciprocal associations with one another, ultimately leading to actions taken or not taken to manage HIV. Every step of the HIV treatment cascade, as well as the HIV prevention cascade, requires youth living with HIV to make decisions to engage with the health care system and/or to modify their behaviors; that is, every step requires active self-management. As described earlier,

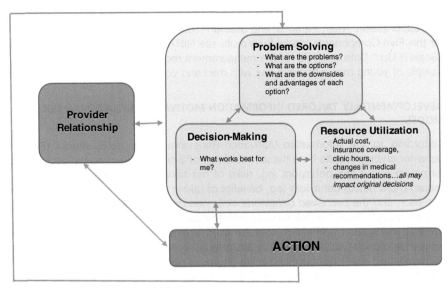

Fig. 2. Five components model of HIV self-management.

few youth actually progress along the HIV treatment cascade from HIV diagnosis to viral suppression.[6,8,9] Moreover, they may be engaging in other risky behaviors such as substance use that interfere across all points in the cascade.[19] In short, these youth are not effectively self-managing their behaviors and not achieving suppressed viral load.

There are many reasons why youth living with HIV may not be effectively self-managing their lives, including impaired problem-solving, decision-making, and/or action-taking. Improved executive function could impact all of these skills positively and may be one important key to improving overall self-management in youth. Executive functioning develops over time as youth mature into adulthood and includes the ability to hold and operate on goal-relevant information in short-term memory, maintain attention in the face of distraction and impulses and flexibly change behavior in response to changing reward contingencies.[72] Better executive functioning in youth is related to better self-control over impulsive behavior, such as drug use and unprotected sex,[73,74] and research in older adults suggests that executive functioning is supportive of prospective memory ability, critical to adhering to medical regimens.[75]

The Five Components Model may be particularly useful for understanding individual-level factors, especially those linked to executive functioning and other cognitive skills (eg, planning, organization) that have been found to impact HIV self-management. However, the model does not extend beyond problem solving, decision making, and the overall contribution of the relationship with health care providers to explain and illustrate self-management. Further, it is not specific to adolescents and emerging adults other than executive functioning and other cognitive factors generally develop and improve over the lifespan,[72] and have been linked to HIV self-management.[76] The model does not include other important influences on health behavior during adolescence and emerging adulthood, such as knowledge of HIV and HIV management, motivation for HIV self-management, influence of peers, and HIV-related stigma. The Five Components model also does not incorporate other important aspects of self-management, namely substance use and sexual-risk-taking behaviors, that have been found to be highly influential on HIV self-management and viral suppression. Naar, Parsons, and Stanton[70] developed a measurement approach for this Five Components model for a multi-site NIH-funded research program called "Scale it Up." Data analysis for the measurement model is in progress for a diverse sample of young men who have sex with men and young people living with HIV.

DEVELOPMENTALLY TAILORED INFORMATION-MOTIVATION-BEHAVIORAL SKILLS MODEL

According to the Information-Motivation-Behavioral Skills (IMB) model (**Fig. 3**), behavior change results from the joint function of 3 critical components: accurate *information* about risk behaviors (eg, risks of not taking ART as prescribed) or their replacement health behaviors (eg, benefits of taking ART), the *motivation* to change behavior, and the *perceived behavioral skills* necessary to perform the behavior (eg, self-efficacy).[77] Thus, the IMB model posits that behavior or behavior change, typically optimal medication adherence, results from adequate information, motivation to adhere, and perceived and objective ability to adhere. IMB has been used extensively to understand health behavior in diverse groups of people with HIV, including adults in the Deep South,[78] adults beginning PrEP,[79] youth starting ART,[80] and people out of HIV care.[81] The IMB model has been the foundation of many HIV adherence interventions[82,83] and has also been used as a theoretic basis in multiple other studies involving youth with chronic health conditions.[80,84–86] Despite this, there are limited studies of self-management behaviors beyond medication adherence, particularly in adolescents and emerging adults living with HIV.

Our group has proposed a developmentally tailored IMB model shown here (**Fig. 4**) to address HIV and alcohol self-management specifically among emerging adults. Self-management is conceptualized as the intersection of core competencies (skills) including self-control, decision-making, self-reinforcement, and problem-solving, and health behaviors including appointment and medication adherence, moderation of substance use, reduced sexual risk behavior, and other general health behaviors (eg, sleep). These core competencies and health behaviors were derived from both the substance use and chronic health condition management literatures. Within this model, improved self-management leads to both viral suppression and better alcohol use trajectories, or reductions in the escalation of drinking over time and into adulthood. The developmentally tailored IMB model also includes information about HIV self-management, including knowledge about HIV and the HIV care regimen, knowledge about alcohol and HIV, and the perceived burden of self-management. The model includes key factors related to youths' developmental stage, specifically youth-specific motivation, or risk perceptions, personal attitudes, personal intentions, social, age-related, and cultural norms, peer values, and stress and stigma. Higher levels of motivation and information are, in turn, associated with better self-management, and improved HIV and alcohol outcomes. Finally, multiple demographic factors such as age, biological sex, race/ethnicity, and sexual and gender identity are proposed as potential moderating factors of the variables and associations within the model.

Human Immunodeficiency Virus Self-Management Interventions for Youth

Most studies of self-management interventions have focused on adults, and the intervention literature for youth is still in its infancy. A recent systematic review[87] of self-management interventions for youth living with HIV identified 12 RCTs that addressed HIV knowledge and beliefs, self-regulation, or utilization of resources, with most conducted in the United States. Intervention response was highly varied and very few

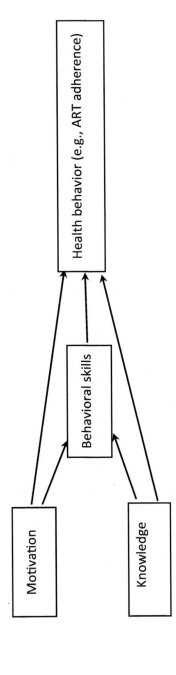

Fig. 3. The information-motivation-behavioral skills (IMB) model.

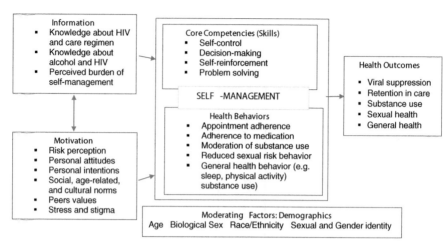

Fig. 4. Developmentally tailored IMB model.

showed effects on viral suppression. For the present article, we identified the few interventions reviewed in Crowley and Rohwer[87] that have shown promise either in full-scale RCTs or in rigorous pilot trials. We also conducted a systematic literature search for any RCTs or rigorous pilot studies fitting the same parameters that were published after the systemic review,[87] but no additional studies were identified. Later in the discussion, we describe the RCTs and rigorous pilot studies included in the Crowley and Rohwer[87] systematic review. These include studies using Motivational Interviewing, supportive accountability, and mindfulness.

Motivational interviewing (MI) is a collaborative, goal-oriented method of communication with particular attention to the language of change[88] that has been adapted for adolescents and emerging adults.[89] MI provides a highly-specified, evidenced-based framework for improving patient–provider communication and promoting behavior change by strengthening a person's intrinsic motivation in an atmosphere of acceptance and compassion. Healthy Choices is a 10-week, four-session manualized intervention that combines MI with personalized feedback on client behavior and goal setting[90] to improve adherence to ART, sexual risk, and substance use in youth living with HIV. In a multi-site randomized trial, youth ages 16 to 24 who were randomized to Healthy Choices plus multidisciplinary specialty care improved viral load at 6 months (3-months posttreatment) compared with youth receiving such care alone.[91] Although in the pilot trial, effects were maintained at 9 months (6 months posttreatment),[92] viral load improvements were not sustained in the larger trial.[91] However, the intervention showed effects on other self-management domains including alcohol use, marijuana use and condom use over 15 months of follow-up.[93,94] In a subsequent comparative effectiveness trial, youth were randomized to home-based delivery of Healthy Choices versus office-based delivery using community health workers.[95] In this trial, the Healthy Choices intervention resulted in improvements in viral load and alcohol use over 12 months. Unexpectedly, the clinic setting outperformed home-based delivery. Of note, participation in the Healthy Choices intervention was also associated with reductions in perceived stigma.[96] Healthy Choices has been adapted for Thai youth[97] and shown to have effects on sexual risk behavior,[98] but its effect on adherence and viral load has not yet been tested in a randomized trial.

The Motivational Enhancement System for Adherence (MESA) is a computer-delivered MI intervention designed to prevent self-management problems in youth newly beginning ART. Two 30-min sessions are delivered 1-month apart and are based on the Information-Motivation-Behavioral Skills model. The intervention is tailored in several ways[99]: (1) youth choose an avatar who serves as a virtual counselor; (2) the interactive intervention is individualized based on MI principles (eg, the avatar reflects participants' motivational language and affirms behave change intentions); (3) participants are routed through arms of the program based on their ratings of importance and confidence, and choices for goal setting; (4) participants receive personalized feedback and ART information based on their recent medical information and response to an HIV treatment knowledge questionnaire; (5) participants may choose to read through the intervention screens or be read to, based on their literacy level and choice; and (6) all intervention content was reviewed by youth advisory groups across the country as well as medical, nursing, and psychosocial providers to ensure appropriate tailoring for the cultural context of adolescent HIV in the United States (eg, age appropriateness of language; appropriateness for ethnic and sexual minority youth). In a pilot randomized trial[80] comparing MESA to a similar computer program targeting nutrition and physical activity in young people living with HIV ages 16 to 24, effect sizes for viral load suppression were medium to large at 3 and 6-month follow-up. MESA is currently being tested in a multi-site full-scale trial. Preliminary outcomes suggest that both MESA and the nutrition/activity control group had significant viral load reductions from baseline, which is expected given these youth are newly starting or restarting ART.[100] Control participants had a significantly greater initial decrease immediately following baseline (and starting ART), but MESA had a greater reduction from baseline to post-intervention (3 months). Analyses are ongoing, but results also suggest that the MESA group may have longer sustained reductions in viral load, out to 12 months post-baseline. Additionally, MESA showed significant improvements post-intervention for HIV treatment knowledge and motivation (as importance + confidence) for adherence to ART.[101]

Belzer and colleagues (2014)[102] found that 3 months of cell phone support calls with incentives for answering calls was so effective in improving self-management and viral load compared with standard care that effects were significant at 3 and 6 months in a small sample of 37 youth living with HIV ages 16 to 24. A sequential multiple assignment randomized trial is underway to detangle the effects of text messaging and cell phone support with and without incentives.[103] This trial is also exploring the impact of tapering, or gradually reducing the number of text messages or cell phone support calls received as part of the intervention.

Webb and colleagues[104] randomized 72 young people living with HIV ages 14 to 22 to a mindfulness-based stress reduction (MBSR) group program or to a health education program matched for format, session number, and length. The 9-session MBSR program included didactic material on mindfulness, experiential practice of mindfulness techniques, and discussions on the application of mindfulness to everyday life. Youth in the MBSR condition were more likely to maintain or reduce viral load than the control group, though self-management was not directly assessed.

To our knowledge, there are no controlled trials of interventions to improve appointment adherence or retention in care. However, one pilot study[105] comparing 2 sessions of MI delivered by a peer with MI delivered by a master's level clinician found both groups to improve appointment adherence 1-year postintervention. Interestingly, the peers achieved even higher rates of MI fidelity than the clinicians, suggesting that community health workers could deliver the intervention with proper training and supervision. Although intervention studies addressing smoking, nutrition, and physical activity are beginning to emerge in adults, to our knowledge there are no randomized trials on smoking cessation or physical activity and nutrition interventions in youth living with HIV.

Clinical Implications

HIV is a multi-faceted disease that creates multiple challenges for adolescents and emerging adults to overcome. Self-management of HIV requires success in multiple domains of health behaviors including medication adherence, retention in HIV care, sexual risk reduction, substance use moderation or abstinence, and general health behaviors such as physical activity, nutrition, and vaccine acceptance. Models of self-management suggest several potential intervention targets. First, having accurate and comprehensive knowledge of the health behaviors required for chronic health condition management and general physical and mental health improvements is a necessary if not sufficient condition. Information should be provided in an interactive way to avoid an "information dump." Motivational Interviewing (MI) approaches suggest providing information in small chunks and eliciting feedback after each chunk.[88,106,107] The teach-back method[108] is another approach to address health literacy and recommends asking the patient to repeat back health information in their own words.

With regards to motivation, MI addresses intrinsic motivation by eliciting and reinforcing motivational language, emphasizing autonomy, and boosting self-efficacy with affirmations.[109] Examples of interventions to boost extrinsic motivation include contingency management approaches (ie, the young person receives monetary rewards or vouchers for abstinence to substance use or viral suppression).[110] Historically, extrinsic motivation and intrinsic motivation were thought to be polar opposites, with the former undermining the latter. However, investigations about intrinsic and extrinsic motivation in young persons have shown them to be separate phenomena, and not inversely related.[111] Targeting both aspects of motivation may have a synergistic effect.[112] Cognitive-behavioral skills building interventions may be used to increase self-management competencies.[113] and may be adapted to mHealth formats.[114] Finally, further research is necessary to develop interventions to manage stress, stigma, and microaggressions, though mindfulness interventions show some promise.[104]

SUMMARY

Although highly treatable with simplified medication regimens, HIV self-management includes complex and related behaviors including retention in care, medication adherence, managing substance use including tobacco, sexual health behaviors, and general health behaviors such as nutrition, physical activity, and vaccines. MI approaches show significant promise in addressing many aspects of HIV self-management in youth, but further research is necessary especially in the domains of retention in care, tobacco use, and general health behaviors. MI-based interventions typically address several points along the proposed frameworks including information, motivation, and problem-solving. However, intervention development around critical components of self-management particularly in the skills domain is necessary to advance the field. Further intervention development to target stress, trauma, stigma and racism, and micro-aggressions is warranted. There are very few studies testing self-management constructs beyond information and behavior. Further research is necessary to test components of self-management and to assess mechanisms of intervention effects across these self-management frameworks. Finally, self-management frameworks were largely developed with samples from Western countries. The applicability of these constructs globally requires further study.

CLINICS CARE POINTS

- Assess the multiple behaviors necessary for the self-management of HIV
- Provide information associated with sexual risk, smoking, and other substance use, and general health behaviors in addition to medication adherence and retention in care
- Use empathic and autonomy-supportive communication to ensure alliance in the patient–provider relationship
- Address stressors including stigma, racism, and microaggressions
- Consider motivational interviewing and contingency management to increase motivation for self-management behaviors
- Find resources for cognitive-behavioral skills building interventions to address core competencies

---

DISCLOSURE

Authors and research supported by grants from the National Institutes of Health (NIAAA, 1P01AA029547) (S. Naar/K.K. MacDonell), NICHD, 1U19HD089875 (S. Naar), and NIMH, 1R01MH108442 (S. Naar/Outlaw).

REFERENCES

1. Kanters S, Mills E, Thorlund K, et al. Antiretroviral therapy for initial human immunodeficiency virus/AIDS treatment: critical appraisal of the evidence from over 100 randomized trials and 400 systematic reviews and meta-analyses. Clin Microbiol Infect 2014;20(2):114–22.
2. El-Sadr WM, Holmes CB, Mugyenyi P, et al. Scale-up of HIV treatment through PEPFAR: a historic public health achievement. J Acquir Immune Defic Syndr (1999) 2012;60(Suppl 3):S96.
3. Fauci AS, Folkers GK. Toward an AIDS-free generation. JAMA 2012;308(4): 343–4.
4. Eisinger RW, Fauci AS. Ending the HIV/AIDS pandemic. Emerg Infect Dis 2018; 24(3):413.
5. Bosh KA, Hall HI, Eastham L, et al. Estimated annual number of hiv infections— United States, 1981–2019. Morbidity Mortality Weekly Rep 2021;70(22):801.
6. CDC. HIV and Youth. Available at: https://www.cdc.gov/hiv/pdf/group/age/youth/cdc-hiv-youth.pdf. Accessed February 22, 2020.
7. Eisinger RW, Dieffenbach CW, Fauci AS. HIV viral load and transmissibility of HIV infection: undetectable equals untransmittable. JAMA 2019;321(5):451–2.
8. CDC. HIV surveillance data tables. Vol 2, no. 2. Core indicators for monitoring the Ending the HIV Epidemic initiative (early release): National HIV Surveillance System data reported through December 2020; and preexposure prophylaxis (PrEP) data reported through September 2020. 2021. Available at: https://www.cdc.gov/hiv/library/reports/surveillance-data-tables/vol-2-no-2/index.html.
9. Kapogiannis BG, Koenig LJ, Xu J, et al. The HIV Continuum of care for adolescents and young adults attending 13 urban US HIV care centers of the NICHD-ATN-CDC-HRSA SMILE collaborative. J Acquir Immune Defic Syndr 2020;84(1): 92–100.

10. Phillips G, McCuskey D, Ruprecht MM, et al. Structural interventions for HIV prevention and care among US men who have sex with men: a systematic review of evidence, gaps, and future priorities. AIDS Behav 2021;25(9):2907–19.

11. Malebranche DJ, Peterson JL, Fullilove RE, et al. Race and sexual identity: perceptions about medical culture and healthcare among Black men who have sex with men. J Natl Med Assoc 2004;96(1):97–107.

12. Pager D, Shepherd H. The sociology of discrimination: Racial discrimination in employment, housing, credit, and consumer markets. Annu Rev Sociol 2008; 34:181–209.

13. Hosek SG, Harper GW, Domanico R. Predictors of medication adherence among HIV-infected youth. Psychol Health Med 2005;10(2):166–79.

14. Bruce D, Kahana S, Harper GW, et al. Alcohol use predicts sexual risk behavior with HIV-negative or partners of unknown status among young HIV-positive men who have sex with men. AIDS care 2013;25(5):559–65.

15. Alperen J, Brummel S, Tassiopoulos K, et al. Prevalence of and risk factors for substance use among perinatally human immunodeficiency virus–infected and perinatally exposed but uninfected youth. J Adolesc Health 2014;54(3):341–9.

16. Elkington KS, Bauermeister JA, Robbins RN, et al. Individual and contextual factors of sexual risk behavior in youth perinatally infected with HIV. AIDS Patient Care and STDS 2012;26(7):411–22.

17. Elkington KS, Bauermeister JA, Santamaria EK, et al. Substance use and the development of sexual risk behaviors in youth perinatally exposed to HIV. J Pediatr Psychol 2014;40(4):442–54.

18. Ritchwood TD, Ford H, DeCoster J, et al. Risky sexual behavior and substance use among adolescents: a meta-analysis. Child Youth Serv Rev 2015;52:74–88.

19. Gamarel KE, Brown L, Kahler CW, et al. Prevalence and correlates of substance use among youth living with HIV in clinical settings. Drug Alcohol Depend 2016; 169:11–8.

20. Williams EC, Hahn JA, Saitz R, et al. Alcohol use and human immunodeficiency virus (HIV) infection: current knowledge, implications, and future directions. Alcohol Clin Exp Res 2016;40(10):2056–72.

21. Williams EC, Joo YS, Lipira L, et al. Psychosocial stressors and alcohol use, severity, and treatment receipt across human immunodeficiency virus (HIV) status in a nationally representative sample of US residents. Substance Abuse 2017;38(3):269–77.

22. Cordova D, Huang S, Arzon M, et al. The role of attitudes, family, peer and school on alcohol use, rule breaking and aggressive behavior in hispanic delinquent adolescents. Open Fam Stud J 2011;4(Suppl 1-M4):38–45.

23. Rosenbloom MJ, Sullivan EV, Pfefferbaum A. Focus on the Brain: HIV Infection and Alcoholism.

24. Scott-Sheldon LA, Carey KB, Cunningham K, et al. Alcohol use predicts sexual decision-making: a systematic review and meta-analysis of the experimental literature. AIDS Behav 2016;20(1):19–39.

25. Hendershot CS, Stoner SA, Pantalone DW, et al. Alcohol use and antiretroviral adherence: review and meta-analysis. J acquired immune Deficiency Syndromes 2009;52(2):180–202.

26. Hahn JA, Samet JH. Alcohol and HIV disease progression: weighing the evidence. Curr HIV/AIDS Rep 2010;7(4):226–33.

27. Clayton HB, Lowry R, August E, et al. Nonmedical use of prescription drugs and sexual risk behaviors. Pediatrics 2016;137(1). https://doi.org/10.1542/peds. 2015-2480.

28. Córdova D, Heinze JE, Hsieh HF, et al. Are trajectories of a syndemic index in adolescence linked to HIV vulnerability in emerging and young adulthood? Aids 2018;32(4):495–503.
29. Scott-Sheldon LA, Walstrom P, Carey KB, et al. Alcohol use and sexual risk behaviors among individuals infected with HIV: a systematic review and meta-analysis 2012 to early 2013. Curr HIV/AIDS Rep 2013;10(4):314–23.
30. Gamarel KE, Nichols S, Kahler CW, et al. A cross-sectional study examining associations between substance use frequency, problematic use and STIs among youth living with HIV. Sex Transm Infect 2018;94(4):304–8.
31. Gleit R, Freed G, Fredericks EM. Transition planning: Teaching sexual self-management. Contemp Pediatr 2014;31(4):16.
32. Valencia R, Wang LY, Dunville R, et al. Sexual risk behaviors in adolescent sexual minority males: a systematic review and meta-analysis. J Prim Prev 2018; 39(6):619–45.
33. Research NIoN. Self-management: Improving quality of life for individuals with chronic illness. 2021. Available at: https://www.ninr.nih.gov/newsandinformation/iq/self-management-workshop.
34. Skinner D, Crowley T, Van der Merwe A, et al. Adolescent human immunodeficiency virus self-management: associations with treatment adherence, viral suppression, sexual risk behaviours and health-related quality of life. South Afr J HIV Med 2020;21(1):1–11.
35. Giarelli E, Bernhardt BA, Mack R, et al. Adolescents' transition to self-management of a chronic genetic disorder. Qual Health Res 2008;18(4):441–57.
36. Arnett JJ. Optimistic bias in adolescent and adult smokers and nonsmokers. Addict Behav 2000;25(4):625–32.
37. Arnett JJ. Emerging adulthood. A theory of development from the late teens through the twenties. Am Psychol 2000;55(5):469–80.
38. Arnett JJ. The developmental context of substance use in emerging adulthood. J Drug Issues 2005;35(2):235–54.
39. Arnett JJ. Emerging adulthood:the winding road from the late teens through the twenties. USA: Oxford University Press; 2004.
40. Parsons JT, Halkitis PN, Bimbi D, et al. Perceptions of the benefits and costs associated with condom use and unprotected sex among late adolescent college students. J Adolesc 2000;23(4):377–91.
41. Chenneville T, Machacek M, St. John Walsh A, et al. Medication Adherence in 13- to 24-Year-Old Youth Living With HIV. J Assoc Nurses AIDS Care 2017; 28(3):383–94.
42. Dinaj-Koci V, Wang B, Naar-King S, et al. A multi-site study of social cognitive factors related to adherence among youth living with HIV in the New Era of antiretroviral medication. J Pediatr Psychol 2018;44(1):98–109.
43. Lall P, Lim SH, Khairuddin N, et al. An urgent need for research on factors impacting adherence to and retention in care among HIV-positive youth and adolescents from key populations. J Int AIDS Soc 2015;18(2Suppl 1):19393.
44. Naar-King S, Wright K, Parsons JT, et al. Transtheoretical model and substance use in HIV-positive youth. AIDS care 2006;18(7):839–45.
45. Naar-King S, Parsons JT, Murphy D, et al. A multisite randomized trial of a motivational intervention targeting multiple risks in youth living with HIV: initial effects on motivation, self-efficacy, and depression. J Adolesc Health 2010;46(5): 422–8.
46. Gamarel KE, Westfall AO, Lally MA, et al. Tobacco use and sustained viral suppression in youth living with HIV. AIDS Behav 2018;22(6):2018–25.

47. Islam F, Wu J, Jansson J, et al. Relative risk of cardiovascular disease among people living with HIV: a systematic review and meta-analysis. HIV Med 2012; 13(8):453–68.

48. Gurung S, Simpson, K.N., Grov, C. et al. Cardiovascular risk profile: A clinic-based sample of youth living with HIV in the U.S. Poster presented at: Conference on Retroviruses and Opportunistic Infections (CROI), March 8-11, 2020; Boston, MA.

49. Masters MC, Krueger KM, Williams JL, et al. Beyond one pill, once daily: Current challenges of antiretroviral therapy management in the United States. Expert Rev Clin Pharmacol 2019;12(12):1129–43.

50. Schlaeppi C, Vanobberghen F, Sikalengo G, et al. Prevalence and management of drug–drug interactions with antiretroviral treatment in 2069 people living with HIV in rural Tanzania: a prospective cohort study. HIV Med 2020;21(1):53–63.

51. Grady PA, Gough LL. Self-management: a comprehensive approach to management of chronic conditions. Am J Public Health 2014;104(8):e25–31.

52. Turan B, Budhwani H, Fazeli PL, et al. How does stigma affect people living with HIV? The mediating roles of internalized and anticipated HIV stigma in the effects of perceived community stigma on health and psychosocial outcomes. AIDS Behav 2017;21(1):283–91.

53. Evans RI, Rozelle RM, Mittelmark MB, et al. Deterring the onset of smoking in children: knowledge of immediate physiological effects and coping with peer pressure, media pressure, and parent modeling 1. J Appl Soc Psychol 1978; 8(2):126–35.

54. Botvin GJ. Substance abuse prevention research: recent developments and future directions. J Sch Health 1986;56(9):369–74.

55. Haegerich TM, Tolan PH. Core competencies and the prevention of adolescent substance use. N Dir Child Adolesc Dev 2008;2008(122):47–60.

56. Lowe SR, Acevedo BP, Griffin KW, et al. Longitudinal relationships between self-management skills and substance use in an urban sample of predominantly minority adolescents. J Drug Issues 2013;43(1):103–18.

57. Wills TA, Walker C, Mendoza D, et al. Behavioral and emotional self-control: relations to substance use in samples of middle and high school students. *Psychology of addictive behaviors*. J Soc Psychol Addict Behaviors 2006;20(3): 265–78.

58. Steinberg L. Should the science of adolescent brain development inform public policy? Issues Sci Technol 2012;28(3):67–78.

59. Chein J, Albert D, O'Brien L, et al. Peers increase adolescent risk taking by enhancing activity in the brain's reward circuitry. Wiley Online Library; 2011.

60. Perrin JM, Bloom SR, Gortmaker SL. The increase of childhood chronic conditions in the United States. JAMA 2007;297(24):2755–9.

61. Fielding D, Duff A. Compliance with treatment protocols: interventions for children with chronic illness. Arch Dis Child 1999;80(2):196–200.

62. Phillips GA, Fenton N, Cohen S, et al. Peer reviewed: self-management and health care use in an adolescent and young adult medicaid population with differing chronic illnesses. Preve Chronic Dis 2015;12:E103.

63. Barlow J, Wright C, Sheasby J, et al. Self-management approaches for people with chronic conditions: a review. Patient Educ Couns 2002;48(2):177–87.

64. Coleman MT, Newton KS. Supporting self-management in patients with chronic illness. Am Fam Physician 2005;72(8):1503–10.

65. Miller AR, Recsky MA, Armstrong RW. Responding to the needs of children with chronic health conditions in an era of health services reform. CMAJ 2004; 171(11):1366–7.

66. Rhee H, Wicks MN, Dolgoff JS, et al. Cognitive factors predict medication adherence and asthma control in urban adolescents with asthma. Patient Prefer Adherence 2018;12:929–37.

67. Amer KS. Children's views of their adaptation to type 1 diabetes mellitus. Pediatr Nurs 2008;34(4):281.

68. Jedeloo S, van Staa A, Latour JM, et al. Preferences for health care and self-management among Dutch adolescents with chronic conditions: a Q-methodological investigation. Int J Nurs Stud 2010;47(5):593–603.

69. Lindsay S, Kingsnorth S, Hamdani Y. Barriers and facilitators of chronic illness self-management among adolescents: a review and future directions. J Nurs Healthc Chronic Illness 2011;3(3):186–208.

70. Naar S, Parsons JT, Stanton BF. Adolescent trials network for HIV-AIDS scale it up program: protocol for a rational and overview. JMIR Res Protoc 2019;8(2): e11204.

71. Health CftAo. Essential elements of self-management interventions. Washington DC: Center for the Advancement of Health; 2002.

72. Miyake A, Friedman NP, Emerson MJ, et al. The unity and diversity of executive functions and their contributions to complex "frontal lobe" tasks: A latent variable analysis. Cogn Psychol 2000;41(1):49–100.

73. Khurana A, Romer D, Betancourt LM, et al. Stronger working memory reduces sexual risk taking in adolescents, even after controlling for parental influences. Child Dev 2015;86(4):1125–41.

74. Khurana A, Romer D, Betancourt LM, et al. Experimentation versus progression in adolescent drug use: a test of an emerging neurobehavioral imbalance model. Dev Psychopathol 2015;27(3):901–13.

75. Hering A, Rendell PG, Rose NS, et al. Prospective memory training in older adults and its relevance for successful aging. Psychol Res 2014;78(6):892–904.

76. Nichols SL, Chernoff MC, Malee KM, et al. Executive functioning in children and adolescents with perinatal HIV infection and perinatal HIV exposure. J Pediatr Infect Dis Soc 2016;5(suppl_1):S15–23.

77. Fisher WA, Fisher JD, Harman J. The information-motivation-behavioral skills model: a general social psychological approach to understanding and promoting health behavior. Social Psychol Foundations Health Illness 2003;82–106.

78. Amico KR, Barta W, Konkle-Parker DJ, et al. The information-motivation-behavioral skills model of ART adherence in a Deep South HIV+ clinic sample. AIDS Behav 2009;13(1):66–75.

79. Dubov A, Altice FL, Fraenkel L. An information–motivation–behavioral skills model of PrEP uptake. AIDS Behav 2018;22(11):3603–16.

80. Naar-King S, Outlaw AY, Sarr M, et al. Motivational enhancement system for adherence (MESA): pilot randomized trial of a brief computer-delivered prevention intervention for youth initiating antiretroviral treatment. J Pediatr Psychol 2013;38(6):638–48.

81. Horvath KJ, Smolenski D, Amico KR. An empirical test of the information-motivation-behavioral skills model of ART adherence in a sample of HIV-positive persons primarily in out-of-HIV-care settings. AIDS Care 2014;26(2): 142–51.

82. Fisher JD, Amico KR, Fisher WA, et al. The Information-Motivation-Behavioral Skills model of antiretroviral adherence and its applications. Curr HIV/AIDS Rep 2008;5(4):193–203.

83. Whiteley L, Brown LK, Mena L, et al. Enhancing health among youth living with HIV using an iPhone game. AIDS care 2018;30(sup4):21–33.

84. Kolmodin MacDonell K, Naar S, Gibson-Scipio W, et al. The detroit young adult asthma project: proposal for a multicomponent technology intervention for african american emerging adults with asthma. JMIR Res Protoc 2018;7(5):e98.

85. MacDonell K, Naar S, Gibson-Scipio W, et al. The detroit young adult asthma project: pilot of a technology-based medication adherence intervention for african-american emerging adults. J Adolesc Health 2016;59(4):465–71.

86. Rongkavilit C, Naar-King S, Kaljee LM, et al. Applying the information-motivation-behavioral skills model in medication adherence among Thai youth living with HIV: a qualitative study. AIDS Patient Care and STDs 2010;24(12):787–94.

87. Crowley T, Rohwer A. Self-management interventions for adolescents living with HIV: a systematic review. BMC Infect Dis 2021;21(1):431.

88. Miller WR, Rollnick S. Motivational interviewing: helping people change. Guilford press; 2012.

89. Naar S, Suarez M. Motivational interviewing with adolescents and young adults. Guilford Publications; 2021.

90. Naar-King S, Wright K, Parsons J, et al. Healthy choices: motivational enhancement therapy for health risk behaviors in HIV+ Youth. AIDS Educ Prev 2006;18(1):1–11.

91. Naar-King S, Parsons JT, Murphy DA, et al. Improving health outcomes for youth living with the human immunodeficiency virus: a multisite randomized trial of a motivational intervention targeting multiple risk behaviors. Arch Pediatr Adolesc Med 2009;163(12):1092–8.

92. Naar-King S, Lam P, Wang B, et al. Brief report: maintenance of effects of motivational enhancement therapy to improve risk behaviors and HIV-related health in a randomized controlled trial of youth living with HIV. J Pediatr Psychol 2008;33(4):441–5.

93. Murphy DA, Chen X, Naar-King S, et al. Alcohol and marijuana use outcomes in the healthy choices motivational interviewing intervention for HIV-positive youth. AIDS Patient Care and STDs 2012;26(2):95–100.

94. Chen X, Murphy DA, Naar-King S, et al. A clinic-based Motivational Intervention Improves condom use among subgroups of youth living with HIV. J Adolesc Health 2011;49(2):193–8.

95. Naar S, Robles G, MacDonell K, et al. Comparative effectiveness of community vs clinic healthy choices motivational intervention to improve health behaviors among youth living with HIV: a randomized trial. JAMA Open Netw 2020;3(8):e2014659.

96. Budhwani H, Robles G, Starks TJ, et al. Healthy choices intervention is associated with reductions in stigma among youth living with HIV in the United States (ATN 129). AIDS Behav 2020;1–9.

97. Rongkavilit C, Naar-King S, Koken JA, et al. A feasibility study of motivational interviewing for health risk behaviors among Thai youth living with HIV. J Assoc Nurses AIDS Care 2014;25(1):92–7.

98. Rongkavilit C, Naar-King S, Wang B, et al. Motivational Interviewing Targeting Risk Behaviors for Youth Living with HIV in Thailand. AIDS Behav 2013;17(6):2063–74.

99. Outlaw AY, Naar-King S, Tanney M, et al. The initial feasibility of a computer-based motivational intervention for adherence for youth newly recommended to start antiretroviral treatment. AIDS Care 2014;26(1):130–5.

100. Hoenigl M, Chaillon A, Moore DJ, et al. Rapid HIV viral load suppression in those initiating antiretroviral therapy at first visit after HIV diagnosis. Scientific Rep 2016;6(1):1–5.

101. Outlaw A, MacDonell K, Templin JL, Naar S. Motivational Enhancement System for Adherence (MESA) for Youth Starting or Restarting Antiretroviral Therapy (ART): Findings from A Multi-site Study. Article presented at. International Association of Providers of AIDS Care (IAPAC), Adherence; March 2020;8-11.

102. Belzer ME, Naar-King S, Olson J, et al. The use of cell phone support for non-adherent HIV-infected youth and young adults: an initial randomized and controlled intervention trial. AIDS Behav 2014;18(4):686–96.

103. Belzer ME, MacDonell KK, Ghosh S, Naar S, McAvoy-Banerjea J, Gurung S, Cain D, Fan CA, Parsons JT. Adaptive Antiretroviral Therapy Adherence Interventions for Youth Living With HIV Through Text Message and Cell Phone Support With and Without Incentives: Protocol for a Sequential Multiple Assignment Randomized Trial (SMART). JMIR Res Protoc 2018;7(12). https://doi.org/10.2196/11183. e11183.

104. Webb L, Perry-Parrish C, Ellen J, et al. Mindfulness instruction for HIV-infected youth: a randomized controlled trial. AIDS Care 2018;30(6):688–95.

105. Naar-King S, Outlaw A, Green-Jones M, et al. Motivational interviewing by peer outreach workers: a pilot randomized clinical trial to retain adolescents and young adults in HIV care. AIDS Care 2009;21(7):868–73.

106. Miller WR, Rollnick S. Motivational interviewing: preparing people for change Guilford. New York. 2002.

107. Miller WR, Rollnick S, Moyers TB. Motivational interviewing. University of New Mexico; 1998.

108. Ha Dinh TT, Bonner A, Clark R, et al. The effectiveness of the teach-back method on adherence and self-management in health education for people with chronic disease: a systematic review. JBI Evid Synth 2016;14(1):210–47.

109. Naar-King S, Suarez M. Motivational interviewing with adolescents and young adults. Guilford Press; 2011.

110. Letourneau EJ, McCart MR, Sheidow AJ, et al. First evaluation of a contingency management intervention addressing adolescent substance use and sexual risk behaviors: Risk reduction therapy for adolescents. J Substance abuse Treat 2017;72:56–65.

111. Lepper MR, Corpus JH, Iyengar SS. Intrinsic and extrinsic motivational orientations in the classroom: age differences and academic correlates. J Educ Psychol 2005;97(2):184–96.

112. Carroll KM, Easton CJ, Nich C, et al. The use of contingency management and motivational/skills-building therapy to treat young adults with marijuana dependence. J Consult Clin Psychol 2006;74(5):955.

113. DAR SON, SER NME. Cognitive-behavioral therapy to promote self-management. Promoting Self-Management of Chronic Health Conditions: Theories and Practice. 2017;31.

114. Cooper V, Clatworthy J, Whetham J, et al. mHealth interventions to support self-management in HIV: a systematic review. Open AIDS J 2017;11:119.

Training Providers in Motivational Interviewing to Promote Behavior Change

Henna Budhwani, PhD, MPH[a,b,*], Sylvie Naar, PhD[b]

KEYWORDS

- Behavior change communication • Motivational Interviewing • Training
- Adolescents • Implementation Science • Communication Science

KEY POINTS

- Motivational Interviewing (MI) is a multicomponent, highly specified communication strategy that can be applied by providers during clinic sessions or in community settings, to promote behavior change among adolescents, youth, and emerging adults.
- Motivational Interviewing training programs should consider inner and outer contexts, alongside bridging and innovation factors, informed by the Exploration, Preparation, Implementation, Sustainment (EPIS) framework.
- The tailored Motivational Interviewing model provides an evidence-based approach to training; it suggests delivery of 10 hours of group workshop training, personalized individual coaching sessions, and tailored assessment based on Motivational Interviewing coach rating scale (MI-CRS) coding of standard patient role-plays or audio-recorded sessions with patients.
- Promoting Motivational Interviewing (MI) fidelity is critical to routinizing delivery in clinical settings; embedding MI into care delivery has the potential to improve youth outcomes across the entire continuum of care.

Funding. Research reported in this publication was supported by the National Institute of Mental Health and Eunice Kennedy Shriver National Institute of Child Health and Human Development of the National Institutes of Health under Award Numbers K01MH116737 (H. Budhwani) and U19HD089875 (S. Naar). The content is solely the responsibility of the authors and does not necessarily represent the official views of the funding agencies.
[a] Department of Health Policy and Organization, University of Alabama at Birmingham (UAB), School of Public Health (SOPH), Birmingham, AL, USA; [b] Florida State University College of Medicine (FSU), Center for Translational Behavioral Science (CTBScience), Tallahassee, FL, USA
* Corresponding author. Department of Health Policy and Organization, University of Alabama at Birmingham, School of Public Health, 330C Ryals Public Health Building, 1665 University Boulevard, Birmingham, AL 35294.
E-mail address: budhwani@uab.edu

INTRODUCTION

Motivational Interviewing (MI) is a highly specified behavior change communication approach to improve patient–provider relationships and care outcomes.[1,2] MI is a goal-oriented style of collaborative communication; in the delivery of MI, particular attention is given to the specified language of change. This MI language is crafted to strengthen patient's motivation and commitment to a behavior change goal by eliciting and exploring the patient's personal reasons for change, which is done within a nonstigmatizing and nonjudgmental atmosphere of acceptance and compassion.[3] MI has been shown to promote behavior change and treatment engagement across multiple behaviors, in multiple formats, and across multiple disciplines.[4–6] Reviews of MI's mechanisms of change have concluded that clients' (patients') motivational statements about their own desire, ability, reasons, need for, or commitment to behavior change (referred to as "change talk") during MI interactions consistently predicts patient behavior change.[7,8] This predictive value, along with MI's emphasis on autonomy support and ability to address apathy toward behavior change, makes MI, tailored for adolescents and youth,[9] an optimal evidence-based approach to scale-up across pediatric and emerging adult care delivery settings. MI is already embedded within clinical guidelines for human immunodeficiency virus (HIV) care and HIV risk reduction in the United States[10]; yet, scale-up and wide spread adoption has been inconsistent. Considering the promise of MI, including data indicating that MI-based interventions, when tailored and delivered with fidelity, positively impact the health and well-being of adolescents and youth, we aim to (1) offer an orientation to MI in pediatric, adolescent, and emerging adult contexts, (2) share examples of MI-based interventions that successfully targeted behavior change leading to enhanced HIV-related outcomes among adolescents and emerging adults that can be extended, adapted, and applied to non-HIV environments, and (3) describe considerations relevant to the successful delivery of MI that are pertinent to researchers and providers, alike. In combination, these sets of information offer a comprehensive primer on youth-focused MI and MI delivery to address health outcomes among adolescents, youth, and emerging adults.

COMPONENTS OF MOTIVATIONAL INTERVIEWING (MI)

Although MI can seem nebulous, it is actually highly specified, includes multiple well-defined components, and incorporates various processes to address a range of patient responses. MI is defined by 3 key qualities[9,11]: (1) MI leverages a guiding communication style that balances following the patient through active and attentive listening and offers direction through the provision of advice and information. (2) MI is crafted with attention to empowerment; patients are empowered to change by eliciting their own personal meaning, assessing importance of the change, and reflecting honestly on their personal capacity for change. (3) MI is based on respect and embraces the notion that patients have autonomy, and that autonomy must be honored. These qualities can balance the power differential between providers and patients wherein the patient's priorities and wishes are honored in the course of their care. In combination, these 3 key qualities inform the spirit of MI.

This MI spirit, a concept central to MI, is informed by partnership, evocation, acceptance, and compassion.[9,12] MI is a collaborative process built on a mutually respectful partnership. Although the MI-trained provider is an expert in behavior change, the youth living with HIV (YLHIV) is responsible for changes that affect their own lives and well-being. MI evokes personal priorities, beliefs, and values to examine why the patient wants to change. MI adopts an accepting and nonjudgmental stance centering on the patient's path to change based on their own experiences and personal characteristics, whereas concurrently respecting the patient's personal autonomy to make decisions and choices. This commitment to centering the patient exemplifies a compassionate approach wherein welfare and well-being are paramount, and the path to change is personalized.

MI is informed by 4 fundamental processes that describe the bidirectional patient–provider conversation flow[3,9,11]: engaging, focusing, evoking, and planning. When engaging, it is imperative to establish a functional relationship with the patient through careful listening and sincere understanding leading to the provider being able to accurately reflect the patient's experience and perspectives while concurrently affirming the patient's strengths and providing autonomy support. In the process of focusing, the provider and patient negotiate a change agenda built on a shared purpose; doing this gives the provider permission to guide current and subsequent conversations into the agreed on direction for change. During evoking, the provider graciously assists the patient to name their reasons for seeking change by eliciting motivations and thoughts. Ambivalence toward behavior change is normalized, examined without critique or judgment and, therefore, has the potential to be resolved. Planning encompasses the mechanisms, or how, of change. During planning, the provider supports the patient to consolidate commitment and craft a personalized behavior change roadmap.

MI, more often than not, is referred to as a method of communication rather than an intervention in and of itself. MI can be used on its own or in combination with other treatment or behavioral approaches. Because MI is multicomponent, including defined processes and core skills, it can act as a framework for behavior change interventions. MI has been developmentally and culturally tailored for youth in diverse contexts.[9] Our group specifically tailored MI for youth HIV contexts using communication science methods to analyze real records of youth–pediatrician interactions in an adolescent HIV clinic.[13] **Fig. 1** illustrates MI's mechanisms of change specifically for YLHIV by demonstrating which provider communication behaviors are most critical in this context.

YOUTH ARE RECEPTIVE TO MOTIVATIONAL INTERVIEWING

Adolescence and emerging adulthood (together included in the broad categorization of youth) is a time of neurocognitive developmental, personal growth, and social experimentation.[14] Youth who acquired HIV through perinatal exposure can become fatigued with their daily medication routine and frequent clinic visits, contend with

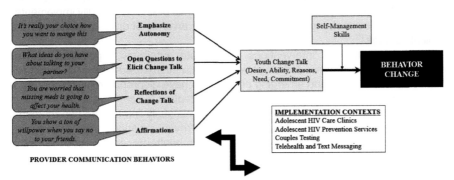

Fig. 1. Integrating communication science, implementation science, and motivational interviewing. (Adapted with permission.[9])

mental health issues, and have to navigate disclosure concerns during sexual debut, and therefore, may respond by reductions in antiretroviral adherence and may resist recommendations from those perceived as holding power and authority.[15–17] Additionally, behaviors that put a young person at risk of being exposed to HIV, such as unprotected sex and substance use, peak during this period. During adolescence and emerging adulthood, poor health behaviors, such as living a sedentary lifestyle and inconsistent self-management of medications, can set the stage for lifelong health problems.[18] Social conflicts with parents, peers, teachers, and providers intersect with biological factors, such as changes in hormones and potentially coping with health conditions, exacerbating the known challenges of this life stage. Because MI is a nonjudgmental communication strategy with built-in autonomy support that is designed to navigate ambivalence, a hallmark of adolescence, MI is a rare framework that has successfully engaged youth to work toward promoting positive behavior change.[9]

Emerging adulthood is a critical period for developing healthy habits in the context of increased cognitive control. The transition from late adolescence to emerging adulthood is marked by anatomic maturation of various brain regions that are associated with cognitive control.[19] Studies suggest that YLHIV, regardless of mode transmission, may at higher risk for disruptions in this maturation process from a highly impulsive state of being toward being more controlled with the ability to weigh consequences of actions; thus, ensuring that YLHIV stay engaged in care is critical to their well-being.[19,20] Considering this transitory development period, approaches that embed autonomy support, such as MI, have the greater potential to keep YLHIV engaged in care as compared with interventions that exclusively deliver content or coaching.

MOTIVATIONAL INTERVIEWING FOR HUMAN IMMUNODEFICIENCY VIRUS (HIV) AND RELATED OUTCOMES

Among YLHIV, MI has indicated positive impact on an array of outcomes including but not limited to reducing substance abuse, promoting HIV knowledge, improving antiretroviral medication adherence, reducing viral load, and maintaining condom use over time.[5,21–24] For youth at elevated risk of contracting HIV, MI has effectively promoted HIV counseling and testing, reductions in substance use, and routine condom use; MI's ability to deeply engage with youth is one of the reasons MI-based interventions to promote PrEP uptake have been developed and are being tested.[5,25,26] To our knowledge, MI is the only evidence-based intervention that has been tested across different points of the youth HIV continuum, has been shown effective in reducing HIV-related stigma (a notable barrier to care), and has been successfully implemented to support behavior change among YLHIV across an array of diverse geographic and clinical settings.[21,22]

Furthermore, tailored interventions to promote autonomy supportive behavior change are particularly needed when working with stigmatized or minoritized YLHIV (including adolescents and emerging adults) who have disproportionally higher rates of HIV infection but lower rates of linkage and retention in care compared with older adults who are living with HIV.[24,27] Failure to successfully link to care and thereafter be retained means that the full benefits of antiretroviral initiation to obtain early viral suppression, leading to benefit in the individual's health as well as reduced risk of transmission, are unrealized.[28]

MI provides a highly specified framework for improving patient–provider communication and promoting behavior change, and high-quality patient–provider relationships are associated with greater likelihood of PLHIV receiving antiretroviral therapy, adhering to regimens, attending care appointments, and having lower viral loads.[21,29,30] Studies have found that MI was effective in demonstrating positive impact across the entire youth HIV continuum of care.[21,29,30] An evaluation of 5 studies on MI's impact on highly active antiretroviral therapy regimens found that most of these studies indicated that MI increased adherence rates; 2 or the 5 studies noted significant decreases in viral load, and 1 of the 5 studies found that MI was associated with an increase in CD4 cell count.[31] Under the auspices of the Eunice Kennedy Shriver National Institute of Child Health and Human Development funded Adolescent Medicine Trials Network for HIV/AIDS Interventions (ATN), multiple MI studies have been conducting with YLHIV and youth who are at risk of contracting HIV; evidence consistently indicate that delivering MI improves HIV prevention and treatment outcomes.[32]

Mechanistic studies of MI show correlations between provider behaviors and patient change talk, defined as the youth's statement of desire, ability, reason, need, or commitment to change behavior,[33] all of which are necessary to promote behavior change for improved HIV outcomes among YLHIV. MI has also been shown to reduce stigmatizing attitudes toward mental illness and substance abuse, conditions that are of particular importance when treating adolescents and emerging adults.[34,35] See **Fig. 2** for an illustration of how provider communication behaviors promote change talk among youth patients, which then influences behavior change.[13,36]

MOTIVATIONAL INTERVIEWING INTERVENTIONS

MI has been leveraged in the creation of interventions designed to improve HIV-related outcomes among youth. Below, we present summaries on 6 examples of ATN-affiliated MI-informed interventions to illustrate how MI has been adapted to address HIV outcomes among youth. Although not all examples have efficacy data from full-scale trials, each offers a unique model of MI. More detailed information on these interventions are provided in **Table 1**.

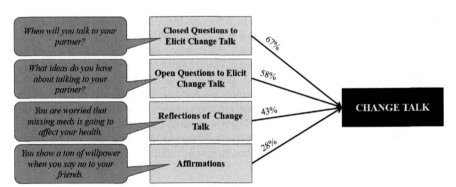

Fig. 2. Motivational interviewing communication strategies linked to patient change talk. Note: Percentages represent the likelihood of producing change talk. "Provider questions phrased to elicit change talk were followed by a patient change talk statement more often than other provider communication strategies. Closed questions phrased to elicit change talk were followed by change talk 67% of the time and open questions were 58% of the time. In addition, reflections of patient change talk (43%), affirmations (28%), statements emphasizing the patient's decision-making autonomy (15%), and information presented in a patient-centered manner (11%) were also more likely to elicit a patient change talk statement. All $P \leq .0001$."[13]

- Healthy Choices,[22,37] based on motivational enhancement therapy (MET),[38] is a 4-session manualized intervention that combines MI with personalized feedback on patient behavior and goal setting. MET was originally developed to address alcohol abuse among adults and was adapted to target sexual risk practices and substance use among adult men who have sex with men who are living with HIV.[5] Healthy Choices has shown to reduce sexual risk, alcohol and marijuana use, and HIV-related stigma while also improving viral load among YLHIV.[22,29,39–41]

- FLEX[23] focuses on the coaching and goal-setting aspects of MI. Developed to concurrently improve physical health and HIV outcomes among YLHIV, while considering the socioeconomic and environmental conditions that limit access to gyms, FLEX includes 3 months of high-intensity interval training, yoga stretching and breaking, resistance training, with self-monitoring and goal settings related to fitness and HIV targets, all delivered in-home with MI.

- SMART[42] tests adaptive antiretroviral therapy adherence interventions for YLHIV. Different that traditional intervention trials, SMART tests a series of layered interventions using an Adherence Facilitator to support the YLHIV through processes. Adherence Facilitators were expected to have proficiency in MI and used their MI skills in all communications with YLHIV.

- Young Men's Health Project (YMHP)[26,43] targets HIV risk reduction and substance use among young men who have sex with men (YMSM). YMHP is a manualized structured 4-session intervention using MI and problem-solving skills building. In the original YMHP trial, master's level therapists were trained in MI with ongoing fidelity monitoring using the Motivational Interviewing Treatment Integrity (MITI) coding system (detailed later in this article).

- We Test[44] adapts and delivers video-based content in a dyadic format with an individual-level single session of MI focused on assisting with identification and development of sexual goals and communication skills. A single-session MI intervention was used because this format was previously shown to have the optimal reach among youth at elevated risk for HIV.[45,46]

- Tailored motivational interviewing (TMI)[47] is the summation of the growing body of work of MI for youth HIV contexts. Although the above described interventions are specified with formal structure and dose, TMI generalizes MI for any HIV-related context, any provider type, any delivery setting or modality, and any HIV prevention or treatment behavior. TMI for HIV has 3 stated goals: (1) Improve HIV-related self-management for prevention and treatment including other related behaviors such as substance abuse and unprotected sexual activity, (2) Provide developmentally tailored strategies to engage young people, considering that the social and emotional needs of youth differ than those of adults, and (3) Train providers from any discipline to integrate MI with fidelity in any setting, from brief 15-minute single sessions to longer multisession interventions.

LEARNING MOTIVATIONAL INTERVIEWING

Several studies suggest that achieving MI competence is difficult for many providers,[48] and that a lecture or workshop alone is insufficient for providers to deliver MI with fidelity.[49–52] Fidelity refers to adherence to an intervention implementation plan, in this case to MI or an MI-informed intervention, as well as competency in delivering MI in scripted practice, routine care, and thereafter for a sustained period of time. Fidelity is discussed in greater detail later in this article. In a study of adolescent HIV care providers from different disciplines across 10 clinics in the United States, only 7%

Table 1
Human immunodeficiency virus interventions that include motivational interviewing

Intervention	Study Participants	MI Trainees	Select Outcomes	Trial Type
Healthy Choices[22,37]	YLHIV aged 16–24 y	Community health workers	Antiretroviral medication adherence and alcohol use	Comparative Effectiveness (for clinic or community delivery)
FLEX[23]	African American YLHIV aged 18–24 y with suboptimal levels of physical activity	Paraprofessionals	Strength assessments, number of push-ups, number of curl-ups, chester step, and body mass index (BMI), with HIV viral load	Proof of Concept
SMART[42]	YLHIV aged 15–24; viral load ≥200 copies/mL, prescribed an antiretroviral treatment, and sole owner of a device capable of sending and receiving calls and text messages	Staff who are not licensed providers but have some clinical training	Antiretroviral medication adherence	Sequential Multiple Assignment Randomized Trial
YMHP[26,43]	YMSM, aged 15–24 y at elevated risk for HIV exposure	Master's level therapists	Substance use and sexual health management	Comparative Effectiveness Type 2 Hybrid Randomized Controlled Trial of the (for clinic or remote delivery)
We Test[44]	Adolescent male couples, specifically: cis-male gender identity; 15–19 y, in a relationship, with a cis-gender male with whom they have or anticipate having sex, and HIV-negative or status unknown	Community health workers	HIV testing and counseling	Hybrid Type 1 Implementation-Effectiveness Randomized Controlled Trial
TMI[47]	YLHIV and clinical providers	HIV clinical providers	HIV cascade outcomes from YLHIV and MI fidelity from providers	Stepped Wedge Randomized Controlled Trial

scored in the intermediate or advanced MI competence range (part of fidelity) using a standardized assessment of simulated patient interactions,[53] although providers reported receiving some prior MI training.

An array of providers may benefit from developing mastery in MI. Studies have shown that clinical providers, allied health professionals, paraprofessional and support staff, as well as community and outreach workers, can all learn and deliver MI with fidelity.[30,54–56] One model found that training youth peer mentors, who were adolescent men who have sex with men, in MI skills was feasible resulting in trainees exceeding established MI fidelity thresholds.[54] What seems to be consistent is that trainees who are committed to learning MI can develop MI skill when trainees are encouraged through the learning process.

Learning MI occurs across 8 distinct steps, leading to mastery: (1) understanding the philosophy of MI (inclusive of collaboration, evocation, and autonomy); (2) acquisition of fundamental patient-centered counseling skills; (3) recognizing and reinforcing change talk; (4) developing the ability to ask about, reflect on, and emphasize statements related to behavior change; (5) reorient one's views toward resistive behavior as a natural part of the change process; (6) hone skills in behavior change plan development; (7) learn to develop commitment from patients to their change plans; and (8) integrating MI with other interventions.[56–58] Learning MI through these sequential steps is time intensive but can be facilitated through a high-quality MI training program that is tailored to the specific needs of trainees and the demands of their work environments.

MOTIVATIONAL INTERVIEWING TRAINERS

Designing an MI training program, standalone or part and parcel of an intervention package, requires thoughtful consideration. Training often consists of some combination of workshops, boosters, and coaching. All components should be led by a senior-level, expert MI facilitator who will be participating through the whole process from design to sustainment to routinization into care or practice. Ideally, the lead facilitator is a member of the Motivational Interviewing Network of Trainers (MINT) so that the trainer is an expert on the most up-to-date conceptualizations of MI. Some experienced MI facilitators are not MINT-affiliated; regardless of MINT affiliation, lead facilitators should be up-to-date and proficient in the most current version or formulation of MI. We recommend establishing a training plan that includes the recipient agency evaluating the proposed lead trainer's MI training experience and if the lead trainer is sufficiently skilled in connecting with the intended audience. The lead trainer may engage more junior facilitators during the process; if this occurs, the lead trainer should be actively involved providing consistent oversight throughout.

IMPLEMENTATION OF SCIENCE TO GUIDE MOTIVATIONAL INTERVIEWING TRAINING

The TMI[47,55] research protocol includes a replicable model for developing a feasible and acceptable training program. TMI is guided by the Exploration, Preparation, Implementation, Sustainment (EPIS) framework[59,60] as an implementation framework to understand the integration of MI into real-world settings. Under the EPIS model, there are 4 phases of evidence-based practice implementation.[60] The exploration phase involves the recognition of a concern or opportunity for improvement. In TMI, the exploration phase includes a qualitative assessment of potential barriers and facilitators to implementation within the inner and outer contexts as specified by the EPIS model. In preparation phase, there is a decision to adopt (and how to adopt) an EBP. In the TMI preparation phase, information about the training on ongoing supports to promote MI learning were developed. During this phase, the team may identify strategies that may overcome barriers to MI training and adoption. Implementation refers to the active integration of the EBP into routine care, whereas sustainment phase examines the continued use of the new EBP. MI training occurs in the EPIS implementation phase. After implementation, trainees enter a sustainment phase; assessment feedback halts.

At each of these 4 stages, EBP implementation is impacted by inner (internal to the organization, eg, organizational leadership, clinician characteristics), outer (external systems, eg, political environment, funding, and other resources) contextual factors, as well as bridging factors (eg, community–academic partnerships) and innovation factors (innovation characteristics and perceived fit for the organization).[60,61] Thus, EPIS represents a set of factors likely to influence adoption and implementation in complex service systems such as those involved in implementing EBPs into HIV prevention and treatment.

TRAINING COMPONENTS: WORKSHOPS AND COACHING

Training components may be delivered either face-to-face or virtually, synchronously or asynchronously, as determined in the exploration and preparation phases of EPIS.[47,59] As an evidence-informed example, the TMI training began with a baseline assessment of trainee competence and skill in MI followed with a 10-hour group workshop delivered by a MINT-affiliated facilitator. Workshop length is variable depending on agency needs but often consists of 5 to 18 hours of didactic and interactive training including presentations, peer discussions, role-plays, reflections, and cooperative learning, spread over 2 to 3 days. Workshop content can include an orientation to MI, in addition to specified modules.

Informed by prior research,[62] MI workshops are structured with cooperative learning activities, video examples, and behavioral skills acquisition steps (modeling, verbal and behavioral rehearsal, feedback). Cooperative learning is a system for teaching trainees in small group settings, using highly specified instructional strategies to encourage trainees to collaborate in teams and work toward a common goal while teammates encourage each other learn.[62,63] Cooperative learning has 3 core ideas that are embedded within instructional activities: (1) group work as a method to enhance individual learning and program retention, (2) positive attitudes and optimism toward subject matter and the learning process, and (3) promotion of problem-solving and interpersonal skills. Studies have demonstrated improved learning outcomes when leveraging cooperative learning.

After the completion of the group workshop, training participants engage in ongoing one-on-one coaching. Based on the TMI model,[47,55] coaching should follow a standardized process: (1) elicit motivation around learning MI, (2) engagement in a scripted standard patient role-play interaction or discussion of an audio-recorded patient interaction, (3) feedback on 2 highest and 2 lowest trainee MI proficiency ratings, and (4) standardized experiential activities targeting the lowest ratings to improve MI skills. Providers should complete 2 mandatory 1-hour individual coaching sessions soon after workshop completion. Thereafter, providers should complete 4 quarterly, brief competence assessments, and receive a feedback report.

TRAINING COMPONENT: BOOSTERS

Booster sessions may be necessary if individual coaching is not feasible in certain settings.[64] Booster sessions engage trainees in brief workshop sessions that are shorter than full workshops ($\sim$4–6 hours) and focus on specific areas of MI skill enhancement.

Although boosters may be preferred by trainees, they are costly and may not lead to enhanced MI competence. In a study on modes of MI training in the Caribbean, researchers found that boosters did not produce a notable increase in outcomes but were viewed favorably by trainees.[64] Booster session, similar to workshops, can be delivered in a range of modalities and can be coupled with coaching.

CODING FOR FIDELITY

Ensuring MI competence and fidelity are critical to success in real-world settings.[65] Fidelity can include individual and aggregated metrics, such as attendance, workshop completion, submitting of recorded sessions, coaching scheduling, coaching engagement, and so on. Fidelity is also assessed via coding of patient–provider sessions. Audio-recorded, patient interactions and standard role-plays are mechanisms to assess competency, and these are evaluated applying a standardized coding scale. Two commonly used scales are the MITI[66] and MI Coach Rating Scale (MI-CRS).[9,67]

The MITI was developed from the Motivational Interviewing Skill Code (MISC); the MITI reduces the length of MISC and focuses on the verbal behavior of the trainee, ignoring patient responses in the coding process.[66] The MITI tool is scientifically reliable and valid enabling use across different settings. Two components are included in the MITI: global variables and behavior counts. Global ratings reflect the coder's overall impression of how well or poorly a trainee performed in a certain element of MI practice, rated on a 5 point Likert scale. Behavior counts capture the trainee's verbal behaviors on appropriate practice of MI.

The MI-CRS has been tailored for young populations and is, therefore, preferred in the context of MI delivery for youth.[67] The MI-CRS consists of 12 items rated on a 4-point scale (beginner, novice, intermediate, advanced) representing essential MI components such as a collaborative stance, autonomy support, open questions to elicit motivational language, reflections of change talk, affirmations, cultural humility, and summaries. To apply the MI-CRS, a trained coder will review the audio-recorded or role-play session and code sections using this framework. Trainees receive an auto-generated report based on scores, with recommendations for practice activities.

Regardless of if the MI-CRS or MITI is used to assess trainee's MI capability, it is important to capture the following elements before the delivery of any training: (1) baseline competence in MI by trainees to measure growth and impact, if any, of training package, (2) identification of which and what (audio recorded or role-plays) samples of MI sessions will be collected and evaluated, (3) determination of who will conduct the coding and assessment, and (4) making a decision on how scored results be reported back to the trainees.

ORGANIZATIONAL FACTORS AFFECTING IMPLEMENTATION

Implementation science is the study of methods and factors influencing the translation of research and other EBPs into routine care.[68] Multiple implementation theories and models have been proposed for the prediction or explanation of the process for adopting and sustaining evidence-based practices such as MI. Determinant models originating from child welfare and mental health fields may be particularly pertinent for the HIV field because of the similar ways in which social context influences program delivery to youth and the adoption of new practices by the clinical care providers.

Our analysis of qualitative interviews with more than 100 providers from adolescent HIV clinics across the United States suggested several organizational factors associated with adherence to an MI training program designed to improve MI fidelity.[47,69,70] Adherence to the MI training program was associated with flexibility in adapting MI to the particularly clinic setting. That is, clinics with high adherence seemed to be more optimistic about the MI implementation strategies fitting into their setting, to have more innovative ideas about handling implementation barriers, and to have a deeper understanding of the EBP and the needs of patients than providers at clinics with low adherence. Clinics who struggled with adherence discussed funding as a primary trigger of turnover and losing staff who had more experience with MI and were more likely to report policy environments that were more restrictive and autocratic in how services are delivered and documented. Clinics with high adherence to implementation strategies seemed to be more autonomous and had greater flexibility with service delivery. They also reported more coping strategies with routine job stress such as maintaining work–life balance and using humor in the workplace. Finally, there are several components of leadership that seemed to be relevant to uptake of implementation strategies including autonomy supportive leadership with buy-in and MI champions at multiple levels of management.

SUMMARY

MI is a highly specified behavior change communication approach to improve patient–provider relationships and care outcomes.[1,2] There is ample evidence to indicate MI's positive effects on HIV-related outcomes among YLHIV and youth who are at higher risk of HIV exposure[21,22,55]; however, ensuring fidelity to MI can be challenging because MI is multicomponent including multiple processes, making it difficult to learn and embed into routine practice.[9,11] We suggest that the TMI model of training, informed by the EPIS framework,[60,61] is ideal for HIV settings that serve adolescent and young adults.[47,55] The TMI model of training includes a workshop followed by ongoing tailored coaching; coaching occurs through the evaluation of recorded patient sessions or standard role-plays, coded using the MI-CRS.[67] To promote the adoption of EBPs, including MI, we suggest that trainings should be tailored to consider organization and bridging factors and inner and outer contexts. The universal inclusion of youth-focused MI in adolescent care delivery settings can make a significant and notable impact on the HIV epidemic and other chronic conditions.

CLINICS CARE POINTS

- Behavior change in resistant adolescents and youth may require multiple motivational interviewing sessions to build provider–patient trust and address apathy.

- The ask-tell-ask technique can be leveraged as a standalone strategy when providers feel stuck in a conversation about behavior change.

- Motivational interviewing training can be as short or as comprehensive, depending on agency needs, priorities, and limitations.

- When assessing motivation and priorities, providers can apply the ruler technique by asking: On a scale from 0 to 10, where 0 means "not at all important" and 10 means "the most important," how important would you say [behavior change] is for you to? Followed by: 1) Why are you at a [their response] and not a [one point lower]? and 2) What would it take for you to go from [their response] to [one point higher]?

- If experiencing hostility toward behavior change, providers can affirm that patient's independence, agency, and autonomy for their own health and decisions.

AUTHORSHIP

H. Budhwani and S. Naar contributed equally to writing and revising this article. H. Budhwani led this study, and S. Naar is a senior scholar and expert in applying MI to improve HIV outcomes among YLHIV.

ACKNOWLEDGMENTS

Research reported in this publication was supported by the National Institute of Mental Health and Eunice Kennedy Shriver National Institute of Child Health and Human Development of the National Institutes of Health under Award Numbers K01MH116737 (Budhwani) and U19HD089875 (Naar). The content is solely the responsibility of the authors and does not necessarily represent the official views of the funding agencies.

DISCLOSURE

No conflicts or disclosures to declare.

REFERENCES

1. Rollnick S, Miller WR, Butler CC. Motivational interviewing in health care: helping patients change behavior. New York: Guilford Press; 2008.
2. Miller WR, Rollnick S. Meeting in the middle: motivational interviewing and self-determination theory. Int J Behav Nutr Phys Activity 2012;9(1):25.
3. Miller WR, Rollnick S. Motivational interviewing: helping people change. 3rd edition. New York: Guilford Press; 2013.
4. Ashman JJ, Conviser R, Pounds MB. Associations between HIV-positive individuals' receipt of ancillary services and medical care receipt and retention. AIDS Care 2002;14(Suppl 1):S109–18.
5. Parsons JT, Lelutiu-Weinberger C, Botsko M, et al. A randomized controlled trial utilizing motivational interviewing to reduce HIV risk and drug use in young gay and bisexual men. J Consult Clin Psychol 2014;82(1):9–18.
6. Burke BL, Arkowitz H, Menchola M. The efficacy of motivational interviewing: a meta-analysis of controlled clinical trials. J Consult Clin Psychol 2003;71(5): 843–61.
7. Gaume J, Bertholet N, Faouzi M, et al. Counselor motivational interviewing skills and young adult change talk articulation during brief motivational interventions. J Subst Abuse Treat 2010;39(3):272–81.
8. D'Amico EJ, Houck JM, Hunter SB, et al. Group motivational interviewing for adolescents: Change talk and alcohol and marijuana outcomes. J Consult Clin Psychol 2015;83(1):68–80.
9. Naar S, Mariann S. Motivational interviewing with adolescents and young adults. New York: Routledge; 2021.
10. Centers for Disease Control and Prevention. Fundamentals of motivational interviewing for HIV 2021. Available at: https://www.cdc.gov/hiv/effective-interventions/treat/motivational-interviewing/index.html. Accessed Decemeber 23, 2021.
11. Rollnick S, Butler CC, Kinnersley P, et al. Motivational interviewing. BMJ 2010; 340:c1900.
12. Hall K, Staiger PK, Simpson A, et al. After 30 years of dissemination, have we achieved sustained practice change in motivational interviewing? Addiction 2016;111(7):1144–50.

13. Carcone AI, Naar S, Clark J, et al. Provider behaviors that predict motivational statements in adolescents and young adults with HIV: a study of clinical communication using the Motivational Interviewing framework. AIDS Care 2020;32(9): 1069–77.

14. Nandi A, Glymour MM, Subramanian SV. Association among socioeconomic status, health behaviors, and all-cause mortality in the United States. Epidemiology 2014;25(2):170–7.

15. Comley-White N, Potterton J, Ntsiea V. The perceived challenges of perinatal HIV in adolescents: a qualitative study. Vulnerable Child Youth Stud 2021;16(4): 320–33.

16. Momplaisir F, Hussein M, Kacanek D, et al. Perinatal Depressive Symptoms, Human Immunodeficiency Virus (HIV) Suppression, and the Underlying Role of Antiretroviral Therapy Adherence: A Longitudinal Mediation Analysis in the IMPAACT P1025 Cohort. Clin Infect Dis 2021;73(8):1379–87.

17. Budhwani H, Mills L, Marefka LEB, et al. Preliminary study on HIV status disclosure to perinatal infected children: retrospective analysis of administrative records from a pediatric HIV clinic in the southern United States. BMC Res Notes 2020;13(1):253.

18. Kim EG, Park SK, Lee Y-M, et al. Factors associated with maintenance of smoking cessation in adolescents after implementation of tobacco pricing policy in South Korea: Evidence from the 11th Youth Health Behavior Survey. Res Nurs Health 2020;43(1):40–7.

19. Mills KL, Goddings AL, Clasen LS, et al. The developmental mismatch in structural brain maturation during adolescence. Dev Neurosci 2014;36(3–4):147–60.

20. Moore S, Parsons J. A research agenda for adolescent risk-taking: where do we go from here? J Adolesc 2000;23(4):371–6.

21. Mbuagbaw L, Ye C, Thabane L. Motivational interviewing for improving outcomes in youth living with HIV. Cochrane Database Syst Rev 2012;(9):CD009748.

22. Budhwani H, Robles G, Starks TJ, et al. Healthy Choices Intervention is Associated with Reductions in Stigma Among Youth Living with HIV in the United States (ATN 129). AIDS Behav 2021;25(4):1094–102.

23. Budhwani H, Bulls M, Naar S. Proof of Concept for the FLEX Intervention: Feasibility of Home Based Coaching to Improve Physical Activity Outcomes and Viral Load Suppression among African American Youth Living with HIV. J Int Assoc Providers AIDS Care 2021;20. 2325958220986264.

24. Hall HI, Frazier EL, Rhodes P, et al. Differences in Human Immunodeficiency Virus Care and Treatment Among Subpopulations in the United States. JAMA Intern Med 2013;173(14):1337–44.

25. Outlaw AY, Naar-King S, Parsons JT, et al. Using Motivational Interviewing in HIV Field Outreach With Young African American Men Who Have Sex With Men: A Randomized Clinical Trial. Am J Public Health 2010;100(S1):S146–51.

26. Parsons JT, Starks T, Gurung S, et al. Clinic-Based Delivery of the Young Men's Health Project (YMHP) Targeting HIV Risk Reduction and Substance Use Among Young Men Who Have Sex with Men: Protocol for a Type 2, Hybrid Implementation-Effectiveness Trial. JMIR Res Protoc 2019;8(5):e11184.

27. Moore RD. Epidemiology of HIV Infection in the United States: Implications for Linkage to Care. Clin Infect Dis 2011;52(suppl_2):S208–13.

28. Ulett KB, Willig JH, Lin HY, et al. The therapeutic implications of timely linkage and early retention in HIV care. AIDS Patient Care STDS 2009;23(1):41–9.

29. Murphy DA, Chen X, Naar-King S, et al. Alcohol and marijuana use outcomes in the Healthy Choices motivational interviewing intervention for HIV-positive youth. AIDS Patient Care STDs 2012;26(2):95–100.

30. Naar-King S, Outlaw A, Green-Jones M, et al. Motivational interviewing by peer outreach workers: a pilot randomized clinical trial to retain adolescents and young adults in HIV care. AIDS Care 2009;21(7):868–73.

31. Hill S, Kavookjian J. Motivational interviewing as a behavioral intervention to increase HAART adherence in patients who are HIV-positive: A systematic review of the literature. AIDS Care 2012;24(5):583–92.

32. Naar S, Parsons JT, Stanton BF. Adolescent Trials Network for HIV-AIDS Scale It Up Program: Protocol for a Rational and Overview. JMIR Res Protoc 2019;8(2): e11204.

33. Söderlund LL, Madson MB, Rubak S, et al. A systematic review of motivational interviewing training for general health care practitioners. Patient Educ Couns 2011;84(1):16–26.

34. Livingston JD, Milne T, Fang ML, et al. The effectiveness of interventions for reducing stigma related to substance use disorders: a systematic review. Addiction (Abingdon, England) 2012;107(1):39–50.

35. Luty J, Umoh O, Nuamah F. Effect of brief motivational interviewing on stigmatised attitudes towards mental illness. Psychiatr Bull 2009;33(6):212–4.

36. Todd L, MacDonell K, Naar S, et al. Tailored Motivational Interviewing (TMI): A Pilot Implementation-Effectiveness Trial to Promote MI Competence in Adolescent HIV Clinics. AIDS Behav 2022;26(1):183–7.

37. Naar S, Robles G, MacDonell KK, et al. Comparative Effectiveness of Community-Based vs Clinic-Based Healthy Choices Motivational Intervention to Improve Health Behaviors Among Youth Living With HIV: A Randomized Clinical Trial. JAMA Netw Open 2020;3(8):e2014650.

38. Miller WR. Motivational enhancement therapy manual: a clinical research guide for therapists treating individuals with alcohol abuse and dependence, vol. 2. Rockville, Maryland: US Department of Health and Human Services, Public Health Service; 1992. Alcohol.

39. Naar-King S, Parsons JT, Murphy DA, et al. Improving health outcomes for youth living with the human immunodeficiency virus: A multisite randomized trial of a motivational intervention targeting multiple risk behaviors. Arch Pediatr Adolesc Med 2009;163(12):1092–8.

40. Naar S, Robles G, MacDonell K, et al. Comparative Effectiveness of Community vs Clinic Healthy Choices Motivational Intervention to Improve Health Behaviors Among Youth Living with HIV: A Randomized Trial. JAMA Open Netw 2020; 3(8):e2014659.

41. Chen X, Murphy DA, Naar-King S, et al. A clinic-based motivational intervention improves condom use among subgroups of youth living with HIV. J Adolesc Health 2011;49(2):193–8.

42. Belzer ME, MacDonell KK, Ghosh S, et al. Adaptive Antiretroviral Therapy Adherence Interventions for Youth Living With HIV Through Text Message and Cell Phone Support With and Without Incentives: Protocol for a Sequential Multiple Assignment Randomized Trial (SMART). JMIR Res Protoc 2018;7(12):e11183.

43. Tanney MR, Outlaw AY, Friedman LB, et al. 159. Adolescent Trials Network (ATN)-Scale it up (SIU): YMHP: Young Men's Health Project. J Adolesc Health 2020; 66(2, Supplement):S81.

44. Starks TJ, Feldstein Ewing SW, Lovejoy T, et al. Adolescent Male Couples-Based HIV Testing Intervention (We Test): Protocol for a Type 1, Hybrid Implementation-Effectiveness Trial. JMIR Res Protoc 2019;8(6):e11186.

45. Bryan AD, Schmiege SJ, Broaddus MR. HIV risk reduction among detained adolescents: a randomized, controlled trial. Pediatrics 2009;124(6):e1180–8.

46. Schmiege SJ, Broaddus MR, Levin M, et al. Randomized trial of group interventions to reduce HIV/STD risk and change theoretical mediators among detained adolescents. J Consult Clin Psychol 2009;77(1):38–50.

47. Naar S, MacDonell K, Chapman JE, et al. Testing a Motivational Interviewing Implementation Intervention in Adolescent HIV Clinics: Protocol for a Type 3, Hybrid Implementation-Effectiveness Trial. JMIR Res Protoc 2019;8(6):e11200.

48. Hallgren KA, Dembe A, Pace BT, et al. Variability in motivational interviewing adherence across sessions, providers, sites, and research contexts. J Subst Abuse Treat 2018;84:30–41.

49. Miller WR, Yahne CE, Moyers TB, et al. A randomized trial of methods to help clinicians learn motivational interviewing. J Consult Clin Psychol 2004;72:1050–62.

50. Mitcheson L, Bhavsar K, McCambridge J. Randomized trial of training and supervision in motivational interviewing with adolescent drug treatment practitioners. J Subst Abuse Treat 2009;37(1):73–8.

51. Moyers TB, Manuel JK, Wilson PG, et al. A randomized trial investigating training in motivational interviewing for behavioral health providers. Behav Cogn Psychotherapy 2008;36(2):149.

52. Moyers TB, Martin T, Houck JM, et al. From in-session behaviors to drinking outcomes: A causal chain for motivational interviewing. J Consult Clin Psychol 2009; 77(6):1113.

53. MacDonell KK, Pennar AL, King L, et al. Adolescent HIV Healthcare Providers' Competencies in Motivational Interviewing Using a Standard Patient Model of Fidelity Monitoring. AIDS Behav 2019;1–3.

54. Bonar EE, Wolfe JR, Drab R, et al. Training Young Adult Peers in a Mobile Motivational Interviewing-Based Mentoring Approach to Upstream HIV Prevention. Am J Community Psychol 2021;67(1–2):237–48.

55. Naar S, Pennar AL, Wang B, et al. Tailored motivational interviewing (TMI): Translating basic science in skills acquisition into a behavioral intervention to improve community health worker motivational interviewing competence for youth living with HIV. Health Psychol 2021;40(12):920–7.

56. Madson MB, Loignon AC, Lane C. Training in motivational interviewing: A systematic review. J Subst Abuse Treat 2009;36(1):101–9.

57. Miller WR, Rollnick S. Motivational interviewing: Preparing people for change. 2nd edition. New York: The Guilford Press; 2002.

58. Miller WR, Moyers TB. Eight Stages in Learning Motivational Interviewing. J Teach Addict 2006;5(1):3–17.

59. Idalski Carcone A, Coyle K, Gurung S, et al. Implementation Science Research Examining the Integration of Evidence-Based Practices Into HIV Prevention and Clinical Care: Protocol for a Mixed-Methods Study Using the Exploration, Preparation, Implementation, and Sustainment (EPIS) Model. JMIR Res Protoc 2019; 8(5):e11202.

60. Aarons GA, Hurlburt M, Horwitz SM. Advancing a Conceptual Model of Evidence-Based Practice Implementation in Public Service Sectors. Adm Policy Ment Health Ment Health Serv Res 2011;38(1):4–23.

61. Moullin JC, Dickson KS, Stadnick NA, et al. Exploration, preparation, implementation, sustainment (EPIS) framework. In: Nilsen P, Birken SA, editors. Handbook on implementation science. Edward Elgar Publishing; 2020. p. 32–61.

62. Millis BJ, Cottell PG Jr. Cooperative learning for higher education faculty. Series on higher education. Phoenix, AZ: ERIC; 1997.

63. Koçak R. The effects of cooperative learning on psychological and social traits among undergraduate students. Social Behav Personal 2008;36(6):771–82.

64. Budhwani H, Naar S. Preliminary Findings from Three Models of Motivational Interviewing Training in Jamaica. Health Equity 2020;4(1):438–42.

65. Allen CG, Escoffery C, Satsangi A, et al. Strategies to Improve the Integration of Community Health Workers Into Health Care Teams: "A Little Fish in a Big Pond. Prev Chronic Dis 2015;12:E154.

66. Jelsma JGM, Mertens V-C, Forsberg L, et al. How to Measure Motivational Interviewing Fidelity in Randomized Controlled Trials: Practical Recommendations. Contemp Clin Trials 2015;43:93–9.

67. Naar S, Chapman J, Cunningham PB, et al. Development of the Motivational Interviewing Coach Rating Scale (MI-CRS) for health equity implementation contexts. Health Psychol 2021;40(7):439–49.

68. Eccles MP, Mittman BS. Welcome to Implementation Science. Implementation Sci 2006;1(1):1.

69. Nagy SM, Butame SA, Todd L, et al. Barriers and facilitators to implementing a motivational interviewing-based intervention: a multi-site study of organizations caring for youth living with HIV. AIDS Care 2021;1–6.

70. Butame SA, Idalski Carcone A, Coyle K, et al. Implementation of Evidence-Based Practices to Reduce Youth HIV Transmission and Improve Self-Management: A Survey of Key Stakeholder Perspectives. AIDS Patient Care STDs 2021;35(10): 385–91.

Resilience-Based Intervention to Promote Mental and Behavioral Health in Children

Yanping Jiang, PhD[a,b,*], Sayward E. Harrison, PhD[c,d],
Xiaoming Li, PhD[d,e]

KEYWORDS

- Resilience • Intervention • Mental health • Behavioral health

KEY POINTS

- Resilience can be conceptualized as achieving positive, adaptive outcomes in the face of adversity.
- Identifying resilience-promoting factors at multiple levels (eg, child, caregiver/family, community) is important to understand why many children thrive despite challenging circumstances.
- Resilience-based interventions show promise in promoting mental and behavioral health of children.
- Interventions focusing on building resilience factors across socioecological systems are likely to be more effective than single-level interventions.

In the past several decades, an increasing body of research has adopted a resilience framework to understand how children respond to adversity.[1–3] As a welcome alternative to the deficit-focused model, the resilience framework shifts the focus of research away from the evaluation of negative outcomes related to childhood adversity and toward opportunities to promote positive adaptation for children and their families.[2,4] From the implementation science perspective, the resilience framework emphasizes the development of positive adaptationother than treatment strategies designed to

[a] Institute for Health, Health Care Policy and Aging Research, Rutgers, The State University of New Jersey, New Brunswick, NJ 08901, USA; [b] Department of Family Medicine and Community Health, Rutgers, The State University of New Jersey, New Brunswick, NJ 08901, USA; [c] Department of Psychology, University of South Carolina, Columbia, SC 29208, USA; [d] South Carolina SmartState Center for Healthcare Quality, Arnold School of Public Health, University of South Carolina, Columbia, SC 29208, USA; [e] Department of Health Promotion, Education, & Behavior, University of South Carolina, Columbia, SC 29208, USA
* Corresponding author. Institute for Health, Health Care Policy and Aging Research, Rutgers, The State University of New Jersey, 112 Paterson Street, New Brunswick, NJ 08901.
E-mail address: yanping.jiang@ifh.rutgers.edu

Pediatr Clin N Am 69 (2022) 795–805
https://doi.org/10.1016/j.pcl.2022.04.009
0031-3955/22/© 2022 Elsevier Inc. All rights reserved.

remedy existing problems.[5] The aim of this paper is to provide an overview of resilience and resilience-based interventions on mental and behavioral health in children.

RESILIENCE IN THE CONTEXT OF ADVERSITY

There is a lack of consensus on the definition of resilience. Resilience was initially conceptualized as a stable personality trait that enables an individual to successfully bounce back from adversity.[6,7] Although the conceptualization of traitlike resilience has drawn research attention, there is no common consensus on what constitutes the individual characteristics of resilience.[8,9] In recent years, some researchers have argued that such a view of resilience as a static attribute fails to consider the importance of the interaction between children and the environment surrounding them in shaping their developmental outcomes.[10] Instead of being viewed as a trait, resilience has been increasingly defined as a dynamic process[5,11] or an outcome.[2] A process-oriented definition emphasizes the changeability of resilience that is dynamically influenced by individuals' internal and external environmental factors.[12] An outcome-oriented definition views resilience as the adaptive outcome in the face of adversity[2] that can be modified, at least partially, by resilience (or protective) factors.[13] Given the focus of this paper, an outcome-oriented definition is adopted to reflect the modifiable and teachable nature of many resilience factors.[14]

The conceptualization of resilience has 2 implicit conditions: one is the presence of significant adversity and the other one is the presence of positive adaptation despite adversity.[11] Adversity refers to a high-risk condition, such as poverty and childhood maltreatment, that places an individual at higher odds of developing poor outcomes.[2] For instance, exposure to childhood maltreatment may be considered a high-risk condition, given that childhood maltreatment has been consistently linked to an increased risk of poor developmental outcomes, including mental health disorders and problem behaviors.[15–17] Positive adaptation can be conceptualized as (1) the development of age-appropriate competence and (2) the achievement of positive outcomes in key domains that are highly relevant to the examined risk.[2,18] For instance, under the first situation, competence for school-aged children can be characterized as maintaining good school functioning over time and may include outcomes such as showing positive adjustment during school transitions, achieving academically at grade level, and developing positive peer relationships.[19] Under the second situation, taking childhood maltreatment as an example, it would be appropriate to operationalize positive adaptation as an absence of clinically significant mental health symptoms,[18] given that childhood maltreatment is a salient risk factor for poor mental health.[15,16] Notably, positive adaptation in this paper is not referred to as superior functioning but is broadly defined as relatively good functioning despite adversity. Positive adaptation, however, is not fixed. That is, children may manifest new strengths and vulnerabilities following the changes in life circumstances as they age.[18]

FACTORS CONTRIBUTING TO RESILIENCE

Understanding the factors contributing to resilience is critical to inform interventions to promote positive adaptation in children who experience adversity. Childhood adversity, such as abuse and poverty, are often deeply situated within the complex family and social contexts that can be difficult to modify quickly. Therefore, identifying resilience factors could guide the development of the intervention by targeting factors known to protect children in adversity against poor developmental outcomes.[20] Resilience (or protective) factors are defined as factors that, when present, can mitigate or eliminate the adverse impact of adversity on child development through modifying how children respond to adversity.[21]

Previous studies have identified various resilience factors that can broadly be grouped into 3 socioecological levels: individual, family, and community.[3,22] Resilience factors at the individual level include personality traits (eg, openness), cognitive competence, positive self-perception (eg, high self-esteem), effective emotion- and problem-solving skills, and high self-regulation. These factors have been indicated to be salient factors in maintaining good mental and behavioral health in the face of adversity.[3,14,22,23] For example, a recent meta-analytic review of the relationship between the "Big Five" personality traits[24] and resilience found that high neuroticism was negatively associated with resilience, whereas other personality traits were positively associated with resilience.[25] High self-esteem, referred to as the positive evaluation of oneself,[26] has also been identified as a key factor in contributing to resilience.[27,28] In a sample of Chinese "left-behind" children (ie, children who remain in remote rural areas while their parents migrate to urban areas for work), children with high self-esteem were found to be less likely to report depression and nonsuicidal self-injury following stressful life events than their counterparts reporting low self-esteem.[29]

At the family level, positive parenting has long been considered a protective factor for mental and behavioral health in children who experience adversity.[30,31] Empirical evidence shows that parental support and warmth may mitigate poor mental and behavioral outcomes associated with adversity, such as poverty,[32,33] war-related traumatic events,[34] and bullying.[35] One process may explain such buffering effects of parental support and warmth on mental and behavioral health within the context of adversity. That is, parental support and warmth may enhance the intraindividual resilience factors discussed earlier, such as high self-esteem,[36] good self-regulation,[37] and positive emotion regulation,[38] which in turn facilitate positive adaptation to adversity. Other family-level resilience factors include stimulating family environments and strong family cohesion.[39,40]

At the community level, social support has been increasingly examined as a protective factor for better mental and behavioral health in the context of adversity.[41,42] The stress-buffering hypothesis posits that having supportive relationships with others (eg, peers, teachers) buffers the adverse effects of stress such as childhood adversity on poor outcomes (eg, mental health problems).[41] Although the evidence regarding the stress-buffering hypothesis is somewhat inconsistent, cumulative studies documented a buffering effect of social support on the association between childhood adversity and mental and behavioral health.[42–46] That is, children who perceived high levels of social support reported less mental and behavioral maladjustment than those perceived low levels of social support.[42,44,46]

It is of note that these resilience factors may interplay to shape children's adaptation to adversity. More recently, building on the socioecological systems theory,[47] researchers have highlighted the importance of the interplay of resilience factors within and across the child, family, and community to facilitate positive developmental outcomes in children who experience adversity.[3,22] With a focus on children affected by human immunodeficiency virus (HIV), Li and colleagues developed a conceptual framework of psychological resilience, proposing that resilience resources within the child, family, and community might work together in a dynamic way to influence positive outcomes, including mental and behavioral health.[3] Such a multilevel resilience framework provides an important perspective on resilience research. Childhood adversity tends to occur together.[48] For example, children who grow up in socioeconomically disadvantaged families may also be more likely to experience other adversities, such as childhood maltreatment,[49] compared with those from high socio-economic backgrounds. These forms of adversity may, in turn, have cumulative effects on children's developmental outcomes.[50] Thus, the presence of single resilience factors may not be sufficient to explain resilience in children who experience multiple adversities.[40]

RESIDENCE-BASED INTERVENTION

A growing body of research has shown the promise of resilience-based interventions to promote mental and behavioral health in children who experience adversity.[51–54] Resilience-based interventions refer to the interpersonal or informational practices that target the building of skills, capacities, and resources at one or multiple socioecological systems to facilitate positive developmental outcomes. The key feature of resilience-based interventions is that such interventions focus on building resilience factors rather than remedying deficits or ameliorating exposure to adversity.[39] Resilience-based interventions assume that enhancing resilience factors promotes an individual's adaptation to adversity and, as a result, reduces the risk of developing poor outcomes later in life or elicits positive changes in current mental and behavioral health functioning. Therefore, the success of resilience-based interventions relies on a solid understanding of adversity (eg, type, duration, chronicity, severity)[40] that the target population faces and the resilience factors that are useful and feasible for individuals to access through the socioecological systems (eg, family, community) in which they reside.[55]

Resilience-based interventions for mental and behavioral health promotion can vary by the intervention content. Based on the resilience factors targeted in the intervention, resilience-based interventions can be grouped into 4 categories: individual-level intervention, family-level intervention, community-level intervention, and multi-level intervention (Table 1). Individual-level resilience-based interventions focus on enhancing intrapersonal resilience factors (eg, positive emotion regulation, positive coping, high self-esteem) to promote children's mental and behavioral health. For example, evidence from a meta-analytic review showed that cognitive-behavioral therapy (CBT)-based resilience-oriented intrapersonal skills enhancement led to short-term effects in improving children's mental health.[56] In another meta-analytic review, CBT-based resilience-oriented interventions were also found to significantly reduce depression, anxiety, and psychological distress in children.[52]

Family-level resilience-based interventions are primarily designed to enhance resilience factors within the home or family environment, such as positive parenting, supportive parent-child relationship, and strong family cohesion, to promote more positive outcomes in children experiencing adversity. For example, some parenting-focused interventions have shown promise in improving mental and behavioral health in children at risk.[57–59] The Triple P, a widely used parenting intervention designed for promoting positive parenting,[60] has been documented to produce both short- and long-terms positive changes in emotional and behavioral outcomes of children.[57] Another parenting intervention—Child-Parent Relationship Therapy[61]—has also been found to result in improvements in children's mental health.[58,59]

Community-level resilience-based interventions are mainly developed to build community capacity (eg, strong community cohesion) and improve access to resources (eg, social support) from outside family (eg, peers, teachers) to promote mental and behavioral health of children. The community environment has long been recognized to play an important role in influencing mental and behavioral health of children.[62–64] Community-centered resilience-based interventions, therefore, have been suggested

Table 1
Types of resilience-based intervention

Type	Intervention Characteristics
Individual-level intervention	Intervention contents are mainly designed to enhance intrapersonal resilience factors that protect against the adverse effect of adversity on mental and behavioral health • Positive emotion regulation strategies • Positive coping skills • Cognitive competence • Positive self-perception (eg, high self-esteem)
Family-level intervention	Intervention contents are primarily designed to enhance resilience factors at the family level • Positive parenting • Supportive parent-child relationship • Strong family cohesion
Community-level intervention	Intervention contents are primarily designed to enhance resilience factors at the community level • Strong social support from peers, teachers, and other community members • Strong community cohesion
Multilevel intervention	Intervention components are designed to enhance resilience factors across 2 or more socioecological systems (eg, individual, family, community)

to be important components of intervention efforts to promote positive adaptation of children who experience adversity.[65,66] For example, Kenyan children left orphaned or otherwise vulnerable, whose caregivers participated in social support groups provided by a local relief group, were found to report significantly lower mental health problems than their counterparts whose caregivers were not the members of the social support groups.[67]

Recently, a growing body of research has highlighted the need to develop resilience-based interventions that target resilience factors at more than one socioecological system.[3,22,40] Although resilience-based interventions focusing on the building of protective factors at single socioecological systems show promise to promote children's mental and behavioral health, some studies have suggested that multilevel resilience-based interventions may produce more sustainable and meaningful changes in children who experience significant adversity.[3,54,68,69] As discussed earlier, single resilience factors may not be adequate for resilience.[40] Instead, resilience factors at different levels may work together in dynamic ways to promote positive adaptation to adversity.[3,40]

Notably, existing evidence, although limited, has shown the effectiveness of multilevel resilience-based interventions on mental and behavioral health in children at risk. For example, the Child-Caregiver-Advocacy-Resilience (ChildCARE) intervention, a multilevel resilience-based intervention designed to improve developmental outcomes in children affected by HIV living in rural China,[70] has been found to produce positive changes in mental health outcomes (eg, depression, loneliness).[54] More importantly, a multiarm design of the evaluation of the ChildCARE intervention provides an opportunity to directly examine the additional benefit of implementing multilevel intervention components (eg, child + family) compared with single levels (eg, child-only).[70] The investigators found that the child-only intervention component had limited effects in improving mental health outcomes, whereas a combination of child and family intervention components led to significant reductions in depression and loneliness.[54] Similarly, another multilevel intervention, designed to enhance coping, parenting skills, positive family interaction, and community integration for families affected by HIV in China, was found to reduce negative problem behaviors among children participating in the intervention.[53]

CHALLENGES FOR RESILIENCE-BASED INTERVENTIONS

There are a few challenges to take into consideration when developing resilience-based interventions aimed to promote mental and behavioral health in children. One of the key issues is the selection of resilience factors that the intervention should target. A good understanding of resilience factors is the foundation of the success of resilience-based interventions.[40] However, this can be quite challenging. Resilience is important for every child, given the high number of youth who experience adverse childhood events and/or contexts (eg, poverty), but there is no "one-size-fits-all" response to adversity. For example, some studies have indicated the importance of considering the potential age and gender differences in resilience factors related to mental and behavioral health.[53,54,71] Findings from the intervention studies have also shown gender and age differences in the effects of resilience-based interventions on mental and behavioral health outcomes.[52,53] Therefore, whether to adopt gender- and/or age-specific resilience-based interventions (vs universal resilience-based interventions) has to be carefully considered.

Also, as presented earlier, multilevel resilience-based interventions may be more likely to produce positive changes in mental health than single-level resilience-based interventions[54]; however, the implementation of multilevel interventions is typically more complicated and expensive in terms of both economic and human resources than the implementation of single-level interventions. Cost-effectiveness analyses may be needed to compare the cost and outcomes between multilevel resilience-based interventions and other types of interventions to make a more convincing rationale for the usage of multilevel resilience-based interventions.

In addition, there is a need to identify the optimal length for resilience-based interventions. Childhood adversities are often chronic and ongoing. Previous findings from resilience-based interventions suggest that a short-term intervention may not be likely to produce long-term, meaningful changes in mental health of children who experience significant adversity.[54,72] Meanwhile, the sustainability of resilience-based intervention may be constrained by scarce resources, as children who experience significant adversity are likely to reside in resource-limited communities.

IMPLICATIONS FOR CLINICAL CARE

Adopting a resilience perspective in clinical mental and behavioral health care calls for recognizing and building on children's intraindividual strengths, as well as protective factors in the home, school, and community contexts where children grow and develop.[73] Although clinical practice is—by nature—heavily influenced by deficit models (eg, evaluating mental and behavioral health symptoms, identifying developmental risk),[74,75] there are important ways that the resilience framework can be adopted in clinical practice and used to strengthen children and families. Adding strengths-based assessment into existing clinical assessment protocols may provide a more holistic view of a child and facilitate the shift of the intervention goal from "remedying" a problem to enhancing factors related to resilience.[73] Gathering data not only on the child but also on the child-caregiver relationship, the broader family context, and other key systems that surround the child (eg, school, social services, faith-based communities) is also important to identify opportunities for positive intervention. Timing effects should also be considered. Resilience frameworks highlight the importance of early intervention for shifting children onto more positive developmental trajectories.[76] Thus, the identification of risk factors (eg, family conflict, poverty, poor school performance) should trigger quick action for further assessment, expanded identification of both strengths and needs, and linkage to positive intervention and support. Importantly, clinicians should also understand that resilience-based interventions have been developed and evaluated for children experiencing a variety of adverse conditions and can be implemented in many settings. Adopting a socioecological perspective to assess risk and protective factors associated with mental and behavioral health is critical, as children's development is embedded within family, school, and neighborhood contexts.[3,22] Providing prompt referrals to strengths-based programs—particularly those that provide support and intervention for both children and their caregivers—is critical for helping children achieve resilient outcomes.

SUMMARY

In summary, the growing body of evidence shows that resilience-based interventions are efficacious in promoting children's mental and behavioral health. In particular, resilience-based interventions focusing on the building of resilience factors across socioecological systems are likely to be more effective than single-level intervention in promoting mental and behavioral health of children, although the empirical evidence is limited. It has been increasingly recognized that resilience is the result of the dynamic interplay of influences across socioecological systems, and therefore, the intervention efforts to promote resilience should consider doing the same.

CLINICS CARE POINTS

- Prioritize resilience frameworks that shift clinical care away from traditional deficit models and toward strengths-based approaches that emphasize the capacity for positive development in the face of childhood adversity.

- Consider incorporating strengths-based assessment in pediatric clinical care to identify intraindividual child strengths and protective factors in home, school, and community settings.

- Develop connections with social services/community organizations and establish effective referrals systems to ensure that children with early risk factors are quickly linked to strengths-based programming.

- Provide education and support for caregivers to help them develop positive parenting practices that promote resilience for children (eg, being responsive and consistent when responding to child's needs, communicating effectively, using behavior management skills).

CONFLICT OF INTEREST

The author has no commercial or financial conflicts of interest to declare.

REFERENCES

1. Masten AS, Best KM, Garmezy N. Resilience and development: Contributions from the study of children who overcome adversity. Dev Psychopathol 1990; 2(4):425–44.

2. Masten AS. Ordinary magic: resilience processes in development. Am Psychol 2001;56(3):227–38.

3. Li X, Chi P, Sherr L, et al. Psychological resilience among children affected by parental HIV/AIDS: a conceptual framework. Health Psychol Behav Med 2015; 3(1):217–35.

4. Masten AS. Resilience theory and research on children and families: Past, present, and promise. J Fam Theor Rev 2018;10(1):12–31.

5. Luthar SS, Cicchetti D. The construct of resilience: Implications for interventions and social policies. Dev Psychopathol 2000;12(4):857–85.

6. Wagnild G, Young H. Development and psychometric evaluation of the Resilience Scale. J ofNursmg Meas 1993;1(2):165–78.

7. Connor KM, Davidson JR. Development of a new resilience scale: The Connor-Davidson resilience scale (CD-RISC). Depress anxiety 2003;18(2):76–82.

8. Maltby J, Day L, Hall S. Refining trait resilience: identifying engineering, ecological, and adaptive facets from extant measures of resilience. PLoS One 2015; 10(7):e0131826.

9. Windle G, Bennett KM, Noyes J. A methodological review of resilience measurement scales. Health Qual Life Outcomes 2011;9(1):1–18.

10. Lee JH, Nam SK, Kim AR, et al. Resilience: a meta-analytic approach. J Couns Dev 2013;91(3):269–79.

11. Luthar SS, Cicchetti D, Becker B. The construct of resilience: a critical evaluation and guidelines for future work. Child Development 2000;71(3):543–62.

12. Dyer JG, McGuinness TM. Resilience: analysis of the concept. Arch Psychiatr Nurs 1996;10(5):276–82.

13. Bonanno GA, Diminich ED. Annual Research Review: Positive adjustment to adversity–trajectories of minimal–impact resilience and emergent resilience. J Child Psychol Psychiatry 2013;54(4):378–401.

14. Chmitorz A, Kunzler A, Helmreich I, et al. Intervention studies to foster resilience–A systematic review and proposal for a resilience framework in future intervention studies. Clin Psychol Rev 2018;59:78–100.

15. Agnew-Blais J, Danese A. Childhood maltreatment and unfavourable clinical outcomes in bipolar disorder: a systematic review and meta-analysis. The Lancet Psychiatry 2016;3(4):342–9.

16. Nanni V, Uher R, Danese A. Childhood maltreatment predicts unfavorable course of illness and treatment outcome in depression: a meta-analysis. Am J Psychiatry 2012;169(2):141–51.

17. Maas C, Herrenkohl TI, Sousa C. Review of research on child maltreatment and violence in youth. Trauma, Violence, & Abuse 2008;9(1):56–67.

18. Luthar SS. Resilience in development: A synthesis of research across five decades. In: Cicchetti D, Cohen DJ, editors. Developmental psychopathology: Risk, disorder, and adaptation. New York, NY: Wiley; 2006. p. 739–95.

19. Masten AS, Coatsworth JD. The development of competence in favorable and unfavorable environments: lessons from research on successful children. Am Psychol 1998;53(2):205–20.

20. Miller-Lewis LR, Searle AK, Sawyer MG, et al. Resource factors for mental health resilience in early childhood: An analysis with multiple methodologies. Child Adolescent Psychiatry Mental Health 2013;7(1):1–23.

21. Afifi TO, MacMillan HL. Resilience following child maltreatment: A review of protective factors. Can J Psychiatry 2011;56(5):266–72.

22. Betancourt TS, Meyers-Ohki SE, Charrow A, et al. Annual research review: mental health and resilience in HIV/AIDS-affected children–a review of the literature and

recommendations for future research. J Child Psychol Psychiatry 2013;54(4): 423–44.

23. Masten AS, Reed M-GJ. Resilience in development. Handbook Positive Psychol 2002;74:88.

24. Goldberg LR. The structure of phenotypic personality traits. Am Psychol 1993; 48(1):26.

25. Oshio A, Taku K, Hirano M, et al. Resilience and big five personality traits: a meta-analysis. Personal individual differences 2018;127:54–60.

26. Rosenberg M. Rosenberg self-esteem scale (RSE). Acceptance and commitment therapy Measures package. 1965;61:52.

27. Dumont M, Provost MA. Resilience in adolescents: Protective role of social support, coping strategies, self-esteem, and social activities on experience of stress and depression. J Youth adolescence 1999;28(3):343–63.

28. Kidd S, Shahar G. Resilience in homeless youth: the key role of self-esteem. Am J Orthopsychiatry 2008;78(2):163–72.

29. Lan T, Jia X, Lin D, et al. Stressful life events, depression, and non-suicidal self-injury among Chinese left-behind children: moderating effects of self-esteem. Front Psychiatry 2019;10:244.

30. Baumrind D. Parental disciplinary patterns and social competence in children. Youth Soc 1978;9(3):239–67.

31. Knerr W, Gardner F, Cluver L. Improving positive parenting skills and reducing harsh and abusive parenting in low-and middle-income countries: a systematic review. Prev Sci 2013;14(4):352–63.

32. Kirby N, Wright B, Allgar V. Child mental health and resilience in the context of socioeconomic disadvantage: results from the Born in Bradford cohort study. Eur child Adolesc Psychiatry 2020;29(4):467–77.

33. Yu D, Caughy MOB, Smith EP, et al. Severe poverty and growth in behavioral self-regulation: the mediating role of parenting. J Appl Dev Psychol 2020;68:101135.

34. Slone M, Shoshani A. Children affected by war and armed conflict: parental protective factors and resistance to mental health symptoms. Front Psychol 2017;8: 1397.

35. Bowes L, Maughan B, Caspi A, et al. Families promote emotional and behavioural resilience to bullying: evidence of an environmental effect. J Child Psychol Psychiatry 2010;51(7):809–17.

36. Growe GA. Parental behavior and self-esteem in children. Psychol Rep 1980; 47(2):499–502.

37. Von Suchodoletz A, Trommsdorff G, Heikamp T. Linking maternal warmth and responsiveness to children's self-regulation. Social Development 2011;20(3): 486–503.

38. Davidov M, Grusec JE. Untangling the links of parental responsiveness to distress and warmth to child outcomes. Child Development 2006;77(1):44–58.

39. Zolkoski SM, Bullock LM. Resilience in children and youth: a review. Child youth Serv Rev 2012;34(12):2295–303.

40. Ungar M, Theron L. Resilience and mental health: how multisystemic processes contribute to positive outcomes. The Lancet Psychiatry 2020;7(5):441–8.

41. Cohen S, Wills TA. Stress, social support, and the buffering hypothesis. Psychol Bull 1985;98(2):310.

42. Wright MF, Wachs S. Does social support moderate the relationship between racial discrimination and aggression among Latinx adolescents? A longitudinal study. J Adolescence 2019;73:85–94.

43. Evans SE, Steel AL, DiLillo D. Child maltreatment severity and adult trauma symptoms: does perceived social support play a buffering role? Child Abuse Neglect 2013;37(11):934–43.

44. Heberle AE, Krill SC, Briggs-Gowan MJ, et al. Predicting externalizing and internalizing behavior in kindergarten: examining the buffering role of early social support. J Clin Child Adolesc Psychol 2015;44(4):640–54.

45. Wolchik SA, Ruehlman LS, Braver SL, et al. Social support of children of divorce: Direct and stress buffering effects. Am J Community Psychol 1989;17(4): 485–501.

46. Henrich CC, Shahar G. Social support buffers the effects of terrorism on adolescent depression: Findings from Sderot, Israel. J Am Acad Child Adolesc Psychiatry 2008;47(9):1073–6.

47. Bronfenbrenner U. The ecology of human development: experiments by nature and design. Cambridge, MA: Harvard university press; 1979.

48. Heidinger LS, Willson AE. The childhood roots of adult psychological distress: Interdisciplinary perspectives toward a better understanding of exposure to cumulative childhood adversity. Child Abuse Neglect 2019;97:104136.

49. Drake B, Pandey S. Understanding the relationship between neighborhood poverty and specific types of child maltreatment. Child Abuse Neglect 1996; 20(11):1003–18.

50. Evans GW, Li D, Whipple SS. Cumulative risk and child development. Psychol Bull 2013;139(6):1342.

51. Skeen SA, Sherr L, Croome N, et al. Interventions to improve psychosocial well-being for children affected by HIV and AIDS: a systematic review. Vulnerable Child youth Stud 2017;12(2):91–116.

52. Dray J, Bowman J, Campbell E, et al. Systematic review of universal resilience-focused interventions targeting child and adolescent mental health in the school setting. J Am Acad Child Adolesc Psychiatry 2017;56(10):813–24.

53. Li L, Liang L-J, Lin C, et al. Changes in behavioral outcomes among children affected by HIV: results of a randomized controlled trial in China. J Health Psychol 2019;24(11):1581–94.

54. Jiang Y, Li X, Harrison SE, et al. Effects of a multilevel resilience-based intervention on mental health for children affected by parental HIV: a cluster randomized controlled trial. J Child Fam Stud 2022;1–12.

55. Graber R, Pichon F, Carabine E. Psychological resilience: state of knowledge and future research agendas. London (UK): Overseas Development Institute. Working Paper; 2015.

56. Ma L, Zhang Y, Huang C, et al. Resilience-oriented cognitive behavioral interventions for depressive symptoms in children and adolescents: a meta-analytic review. J affective Disord 2020;270:150–64.

57. Sanders MR, Kirby JN, Tellegen CL, et al. The Triple P-positive parenting program: a systematic review and meta-analysis of a multi-level system of parenting support. Clin Psychol Rev 2014;34(4):337–57.

58. Ceballos PL, Lin Y-W, Bratton SC, et al. Effects of parenting programs on Latina mothers' parental stress and their children's internalizing behavioral problems. J child Adolesc Couns 2019;5(1):73–88.

59. Dillman Taylor D, Purswell K, Lindo N, et al. The impact of child parent relationship therapy on child behavior and parent-child relationships: An examination of parental divorce. Int J Play Ther 2011;20(3):124.

60. Sanders MR. Triple P-Positive Parenting Program as a public health approach to strengthening parenting. J Fam Psychol 2008;22(4):506.

61. Bratton SC, Landreth GL. Child parent relationship therapy (CPRT) treatment manual: a 10-session filial therapy model for training parents. New York, NY: Routledge; 2006.
62. Goodman A, Fleitlich-Bilyk B, Patel V, et al. Child, family, school and community risk factors for poor mental health in Brazilian schoolchildren. J Am Acad Child Adolesc Psychiatry 2007;46(4):448–56.
63. Trach J, Lee M, Hymel S. A social-ecological approach to addressing emotional and behavioral problems in schools: focusing on group processes and social dynamics. J Emotional Behav Disord 2018;26(1):11–20.
64. Baker JA, Grant S, Morlock L. The teacher-student relationship as a developmental context for children with internalizing or externalizing behavior problems. Sch Psychol Q 2008;23(1):3.
65. Wessells M. Strengths-based community action as a source of resilience for children affected by armed conflict. Glob Ment Health 2016;3:e1.
66. Barry MM, Clarke AM, Jenkins R, et al. A systematic review of the effectiveness of mental health promotion interventions for young people in low and middle income countries. BMC Public health 2013;13(1):1–19.
67. Thurman TR, Jarabi B, Rice J. Caring for the caregiver: evaluation of support groups for guardians of orphans and vulnerable children in Kenya. AIDS care 2012;24(7):811–9.
68. Harrison S, Li X. Rebooting resilience: shifts toward dynamic, multi-level, and technology-based approaches for people living with HIV. AIDS care 2018; 30(suppl 5):S1–5.
69. Cicchetti D. Resilience under conditions of extreme stress: a multilevel perspective. World Psychiatry 2010;9(3):145.
70. Li X, Harrison SE, Fairchild AJ, et al. A randomized controlled trial of a resilience-based intervention on psychosocial well-being of children affected by HIV/AIDS: Effects at 6-And 12-month Follow-Up. Social Sci Med (1982) 2017;190:256–64.
71. Sun J, Stewart D. Age and gender effects on resilience in children and adolescents. Int J Ment Health Promot 2007;9(4):16–25.
72. Jiang Y, Li X, Harrison SE, et al. Long-term effects of a resilience-based intervention on mental health of children affected by parental HIV in China: Testing the mediation effects of emotion regulation and coping. Child Youth Serv Rev 2022;133:106363.
73. Tedeschi RG, Kilmer RP. Assessing strengths, resilience, and growth to guide clinical interventions. Prof Psychol Res Pract 2005;36(3):230.
74. Szmukler G, Rose N. Risk assessment in mental health care: Values and costs. Behav Sci Law 2013;31(1):125–40.
75. Crowe M, Carlyle D. Deconstructing risk assessment and management in mental health nursing. J Adv Nurs 2003;43(1):19–27.
76. Sapienza JK, Masten AS. Understanding and promoting resilience in children and youth. Curr Opin Psychiatry 2011;24(4):267–73.

Behavioral Intervention for Nonmedical Use of Prescription Drugs Among Adolescents and Young Adults
A Narrative Review

Cheuk Chi Tam, PhD[a], Shelby A. Smout, MS[b],
Catherine S.J. Wall, BS[b], Kyle Liam Mason, MS[b],
Eric G. Benotsch, PhD[b],*

KEYWORDS

- Nonmedical use of prescription drugs • Intervention • Adolescents • Young adults
- Opioids

KEY POINTS

- Primary prevention interventions have proven to be effective in reducing positive expectancies about nonmedical use of prescription drugs (NMUPD) and in increasing knowledge about NMUPD across individual, group, and community level interventions.
- Both in-person and technology-facilitated interventions have shown promise in reducing NMUPD in adolescents and young adults.
- The interventions with the greatest demonstrated efficacy are interventions that involve parent-child dyads, which were associated with lower NMUPD and other forms of substance use at follow-up.
- Most current NMUPD interventions focus on primary prevention (ie, universal and selective prevention) with few focusing on secondary prevention.
- Few studies take a multilevel (individual, group, and community) approach to NMUPD interventions, which has been successfully used to address other forms of substance use among adolescents and young adults.

The nonmedical use of prescription drugs (NMUPD) refers to the use of prescription drugs typically used for managing pain or treating psychiatric conditions that were not prescribed for the individual by a physician or are used only for the experience

---

[a] South Carolina SmartState Center for Healthcare Quality, Department of Health Promotion, Education, and Behavior, Arnold School of Public Health, University of South Carolina, 915 Green Street, Columbia, SC 29208, USA; [b] Department of Psychology, Virginia Commonwealth University, 806 West Franklin Street, Box 842018, Richmond, VA 23284-2018, USA
* Corresponding author.
E-mail address: ebenotsch@vcu.edu

Pediatr Clin N Am 69 (2022) 807–818
https://doi.org/10.1016/j.pcl.2022.04.010
0031-3955/22/© 2022 Elsevier Inc. All rights reserved.

or feeling they cause.[1] Common nonmedically used prescription drugs include opioids (eg, Oxycodone), anxiolytics (eg, Lorazepam), sedatives (eg, Zolpidem), and stimulants (eg, methylphenidate). In the United States, NMUPD is a critical public health problem owing to its detrimental impacts, including large numbers of overdose deaths (eg, >60,000 annually),[2] emergency department visits (eg, 358,247 in 2016),[3] and extensive economic burden (estimated cost of $78.5 billion in 2013).[4] Overall, young adults and adolescents are the age groups most likely to engage in NMUPD.[5] Notably, recent data have shown that many US young people initiated NMUPD in the past year, including 290,000 young adults and 158,000 adolescents engaged in nonmedical use of opioids, 290,000 young adults and 103,000 adolescents engaged in nonmedical use of anxiolytics, and 18,000 young adults and 77,000 adolescents engaged in nonmedical use of sedatives for the first time.[5]

Engagement in NMUPD among adolescents and young adults is associated with detrimental physical and psychological consequences, including drug dependence and abuse,[6] initiation of other substance use,[6] polysubstance use,[7] injection-related infections,[8] and nonfatal and fatal overdoses.[2] NMUPD is also associated with other risk behaviors, including high-risk sex and driving under the influence of prescription drugs used nonmedically.[9,10] Adolescents and young adults who engage in NMUPD also experience social consequences, including difficulties in academic settings, such as missing classes and lower grades.[11]

Substance use interventions can be delivered at multiple levels, including individual, families, or other groups (eg, classrooms), and at the broader community level. Each of these approaches has advantages. Individual level interventions, for example, are the easiest to tailor to individual needs. Interventions delivered to small groups can enlist aspects of group/family dynamics as part of the treatment process. Community interventions can affect large numbers of individuals and can influence norms.[12] Each of these approaches has been used in interventions designed to reduce NMUPD among adolescents and young adults.

Although many interventions continue to be conducted in person, researchers and clinicians are also increasingly using technology to deliver interventions to prevent NMUPD. Internet and other technology-facilitated interventions have been shown to be effective in decreasing substance use.[13,14] The high utilization of technology among adolescents and young adults may increase the possibility of accessing needed interventions; however, differences in Internet access based in economic inequality and regional divides may impact intervention accessibility while furthering disparities based in intergroup inequality. Although Internet-based interventions are invaluable in a technologically savvy world, they may still remain out of reach for certain at-risk populations.[15]

The goal of this narrative review is to describe recent prevention interventions for NMUPD that were directed at adolescents and young adults. The authors include interventions directed to individuals, small groups and families, and communities and include both in-person and technology-facilitated interventions. Both randomized controlled trials (RCT) and single group designs were included. To identify studies, the authors searched PsycINFO, PubMed, Web of Science, and Google Scholar. An additional search was conducted using the general Google search function to identify research not reported in an academic journal. Studies were selected and reviewed if they met all of the following criteria: (1) interventions directed at adolescents or young adults (ages 12–25); (2) interventions conducted in the United States; (3) interventions directed at the use of substances, including NMUPD; (4) studies reporting some outcome data related to either NMUPD or cognitive/psychological mediators theorized to predicted NMUPD (eg, NMUPD intentions); (5) studies conducted between

1980 and 2021. Findings of the reviewed studies were then reported and organized in line with the intervention classification guided by the Institute of Medicine (IOM) framework.[16,17]

RESULTS

According to the IOM framework,[16,17] the reviewed studies were identified as primary prevention interventions, which targeted adolescents or young adults without a history or detected occurrence of NMUPD. In terms of their prevention strategies, the reviewed studies were categorized into universal prevention (targeting general samples of adolescents or young adults) and selective prevention (targeting adolescent or young adults who were at increased risk for NMUPD). Each category included interventions using in-person meetings or technology directed at the individual level, family or group level, and community level. The search strategy did not identify any secondary prevention interventions (ie, interventions delivered to adolescents or young adults who were already engaged in NMUPD) that met inclusion criteria.

Universal Prevention

Technology-facilitated interventions directed at the individual level
Arabyat and colleagues[18] recruited 391 college students to participate in an RCT with immediate postintervention assessment only. Intervention participants received an online intervention based on the reasoned action approach[19] that included elements aimed at changing attitudes, perceived norms, perceived behavioral control, and intentions. Techniques included providing participants with accurate information about the effects of NMUPD (attitudes) and the prevalence of NMUPD (norms), as well as increasing self-efficacy of participants to avoid NMUPD (perceived behavioral control). To increase engagement, audio and video components, interactive tools, and a quiz were included. Control group participants viewed a general health Web site. At the postassessment, intervention participants had more negative attitudes toward NMUPD than participants in the control group. There were no differences between the 2 groups in perceived norms, perceived behavioral control, or intentions to engage in NMUPD.

Marsch and colleagues[20] conducted an RCT with 406 adolescents (ages 12–17) designed to reduce nonmedical use of opioids. The newly created intervention, Pop4Teens, was compared with an existing intervention, Just Think Twice, that is run by the US Drug Enforcement Agency. Both interventions were delivered online. The Pop4Teens intervention focused on increasing knowledge about the risk of nonmedical use of opioids and improving drug refusal skills. To increase engagement, the Pop4Teens intervention used a storytelling component (stories from real teens in recovery from opioid abuse), an educational component, a skill-based video, and a quiz. Participants were asked to complete 8 modules over the course of 4 weeks. The Just Think Twice intervention is a publicly available Web site that provides education for teens about the use of opioids and other substances and strategies to avoid use. Participants in this arm were asked to use the Just Think Twice Web site twice per week for 4 weeks. Both interventions resulted in increases in perceived risk of nonmedical use of opioids, reductions in positive expectancies regarding opioid use, increases in self-efficacy for opioid refusal, and reductions in intentions to use opioids. Pop4Teens participants had significantly greater improvements in opioid-related knowledge than Just Think Twice participants, and the Pop4Teen intervention was perceived as easier to use. Participants' actual use of opioids was not assessed.

Interventions directed at the family or group level via in person meetings

Carson[21] conducted a quasi-experimental trial with adolescents (N = 318; mean age = 15 years) attending schools in Indiana. Intervention schools received the "This is Not About Drugs" (TINAD) intervention, and control schools were assigned to a wait list for the same intervention. TINAD focused primarily on education regarding opioids, including both heroin use and the nonmedical use of prescription opioids, and sought to improve understanding of the risks of opioid use and to increase use of adaptive coping strategies. The intervention was delivered at the classroom level. Using a pre-post design, students receiving TINAD showed significant increases in the perceived risk of nonmedical use of opioids and greater knowledge of some aspects of opioid use; however, there were no significant changes in coping strategies.

Evans and colleagues[22] conducted a second test of the TINAD program in middle school students (N = 576; mean age = 11.8 years) in one rural county in the southeastern United States. Immediately following intervention delivery, participants scored higher on measures assessing knowledge about nonmedical use of opioids, perceived severity of nonmedical use of opioids, and increased self-efficacy for avoiding nonmedical use of opioids. There was no change in intentions to use opioids nonmedically; however, this may have been due to a floor effect, as most participants at pretest reported low intentions to engage in the nonmedical use of opioids.

Patry and colleagues[23] recruited ninth graders in 8 Rhode Island high schools to receive an educational intervention about the risks of nonmedical use of opioids. The intervention was delivered by pharmacy students in classroom settings over 3 to 4 sessions of around 1 hour each and included didactic portions as well as interactive role-plays. In this pre-post design, adolescents at the postintervention assessment had higher knowledge regarding the risks of nonmedical use of opioids. They also reported greater confidence in identifying the signs of an opioid overdose, knowing when to refer someone to treatment, and knowing when to administer naloxone for opioid overdose.

Spoth and colleagues[24] reported on the long-term follow-up of an RCT conducted in Iowa schools in 1993. The trial targeted substance use but not NMUPD specifically. The study recruited 667 sixth graders and randomly assigned them to the following: (1) Iowa Strengthening Families Program; (2) Preparing for Drug Free Years; or (3) control condition. The Iowa Strengthening Families Program is a 7-session program with adolescents and their parents focused on family risk and protective factors. Parents received education on nurturing, communication skills, and child management skills. Adolescents received education on resisting peer pressure, managing conflict, and developing healthy friendships. Some sessions were specifically for parents; others were specifically for the adolescents, and some were family sessions in which all participants attended. The Preparing for Drug Free Years intervention is delivered over 5 sessions. One session is specifically for the adolescent and focuses on resisting peer pressure and drug refusal skills. The other 4 sessions are for the parents and focus on family management, communication skills, and parent-child bonding. NMUPD was not assessed at baseline, but a question about nonmedical use of opioids was added for the 12th grade follow-up. Results showed that significantly fewer adolescents receiving the Iowa Strengthening Families Program reported nonmedical use of opioids at the 12th grade follow-up when compared with the control condition. There was a nonsignificant effect for the Preparing for Drug Free Years program (P = .07).

In 1998, Spoth and colleagues[25] modified the intervention components and conducted a second RCT with 2127 seventh graders and randomly assigned them to the following: (1) Life Skills training program; (2) modified version of the Iowa Strengthening Families Program; or (3) control condition. In this study, the Life Skills intervention consists of 15 sessions of around 45 minutes each taught by teachers during the school day. An additional 5 booster sessions were presented 1 year later for all participants, and half of the intervention participants were randomly assigned to receive an additional 5 booster sessions 4 years after the initial intervention. The modified version of the Iowa Strengthening Families Program (now called the Strengthening Families Program: For Parents and Youth 10–14 [SFP: 10–14]) focused on the same material as the original version but was adapted to include more interactive features, such as games, and intervention components were presented in a different order. Similar to the first study, NMUPD was not assessed at baseline, but a question was administered at both 11th and 12th grade that asked about the use of prescription medications not prescribed to the individual. Results showed that at the 11th grade assessment, significantly fewer participants receiving the SFP: 10 to 14 intervention reported NMUPD than controls; this difference was nonsignificant ($P = .061$) at the 12th grade follow-up. Participants receiving the Life Skills program were less likely to report NMUPD than the controls at both times points, but neither difference was statistically significant. Spoth and colleagues[25] reported longer-term follow-up for the first and second trials when participants were 25 years of age (study 1) and 21, 22, and 25 years of age (study 2). In general, participants in the Iowa Strengthening Families Program/SFP: 10 to 14, conditions continued to report lower rates of NMUPD than participants in the control conditions.

Spoth and colleagues[26] also reported outcomes from a third RCT conducted with more than 10,000 sixth to seventh graders recruited from 28 rural school districts in Iowa and Pennsylvania. Schools involved in this trial were offered both the SFP: 10 to 14 intervention (delivered in sixth grade) and 1 of 3 school-based interventions (All Stars, Life Skills, Project Alert) delivered in seventh grade that focused on increasing accuracy of peer norms for NMUPD, resisting peer pressure, and drug refusal skills, versus a control condition. Only 17% of eligible families participated in SFP: 10 to 14; however, almost all eligible adolescents received the school-based programs. Intervention participants completing a follow-up assessment in 12th grade reported significantly less NMUPD than control participants. In an additional analysis of this trial, Crowley and colleagues[27] reported that participants receiving SFP: 10 to 14 coupled with either the All Stars or Life Skills school-based interventions reported significantly less NMUPD than control participants. Furthermore, participants who received the Life Skills intervention alone reported significantly less NMUPD than control participants. Each of these interventions was also cost-effective.[27]

Technology-facilitated interventions directed at the family or group level
Fang and colleagues[28] recruited 108 Asian American girls (ages 10–14) and their mothers for a family intervention directed at caregiver-child dyads. Dyads were randomly assigned to an intervention or no-treatment control arm. Intervention dyads received a 9-week online intervention based on family interaction theory. The intervention used voice-over animation, graphics, skill demonstrations, and games to deliver content designed to improve mother-daughter communication, maternal monitoring, daughters' mental health and drug refusal skills, and to reduce substance use intentions and substance use among the daughters. Each session lasted around 45 minutes. At 6-month follow-up, adolescent girls assigned to the intervention condition, relative to controls, reported less depressed mood, greater closeness to their mothers, better mother-daughter communication, increased maternal monitoring, greater drug refusal skills, and lower substance use intentions. In addition, girls assigned to the intervention condition reported significantly less NMUPD as well as less use of alcohol and cannabis, relative to girls assigned to the control condition.

A 2-year follow-up with the same participants indicated that intervention daughters had sustained improvement in mood, closeness to their mothers, mother-daughter communication, maternal monitoring, drug refusal skills, and lower substance use intentions.[29] They also reported significantly lower NMUPD and use of alcohol and cannabis relative to daughters in the control condition.

Schinke and colleagues[30] recruited 591 adolescent girls (mean age = 12.6 years) and their mothers from New York, New Jersey, and Connecticut to conduct an RCT comparing a gender-specific computer-based intervention aimed at preventing substance use to a no treatment control group. Participants completed nine 45-minute sessions that focused on improving communication, increasing daughters' self-esteem, communicating family rules and consequences related to substance use, and increasing daughters' self-efficacy, stress management, and peer pressure refusal skills. Elements of the intervention included voice-over narration, skills demonstrations, and interactive exercises completed jointly by mothers and daughters. At 1-year follow-up, adolescent girls in the intervention condition were significantly less likely to report the use of alcohol, cannabis, or NMUPD than girls in the control condition. Intervention participants also reported better communication, greater understanding of family rules, greater drug refusal skills, and lower intentions to use substances. Schinke and colleagues[31] reported data from a 2-year follow-up of this study in which an additional 325 mother-daughter dyads were enrolled. Results showed that at 2 years, girls in the intervention condition were significantly less likely to report the use of alcohol, cannabis, inhalants, or NMUPD and continued to score higher on protective factors (eg, communication) than girls in the control condition. Mothers in the intervention condition also reported lower rates of weekly alcohol consumption than control condition mothers.

Community level interventions delivered in person

Johnson and colleagues,[32] Ogilvie and colleagues,[33] Gruenewald and colleagues,[34] and Courser and colleagues[35] describe a multipronged intervention delivered at both the community and the group level to reduce the misuse of harmful legal products, including prescription drugs, over-the-counter medications, and inhalants, among adolescents (grades 5–7) in 3 rural Alaskan communities. Community aspects of the intervention included making retailers aware of how adolescents can use products for the purposes of intoxication, developing store policies restricting the sale of these products to minors, and storing such products behind the counter. Home-based strategies included educating parents about products that are used by adolescents for the purpose of intoxication and encouraging restricting access to those products by placing prescription medications in a locked cabinet. School-based strategies were also implemented to reduce misuse of cleaning products or art supplies. At the group level, the ThinkSmart intervention was delivered to fifth graders in these communities. ThinkSmart is a 15-hour intervention delivered in health classes that focuses on increasing knowledge of the risks of harmful legal products, including prescription drugs used nonmedically and to improve drug refusal skills. At follow-up, adolescents in this single group study had higher knowledge of the risks of harmful legal products and perceived these products as less available in their community when compared with their baseline scores.[36] In addition, parents and school officials reported taking actions to reduce access to potentially abusable substances.[34] Furthermore, the project implemented youth (ages 12–17) purchase attempts of potentially harmful substances at community retailers and reported a significant reduction in successful purchases from baseline to follow-up.[35]

Selective Prevention

Interventions directed at the individual level via in person meetings

Looby and colleagues[36] recruited 96 college students who had never engaged in NMUPD, but were perceived to be at high risk of doing so because of having a low grade point average, being a member of a Greek organization (ie, fraternity, sorority), or having recent high-risk use of alcohol or cannabis. Participants were randomly assigned to the intervention or a no-treatment control condition. Intervention participants were asked to ingest a placebo pill but were told that it was methylphenidate, a prescription stimulant. Later, intervention participants were debriefed and told that they had actually received a placebo. The intent with this procedure was to demonstrate to participants that any perceived changes in their cognitive functioning were the result of expectancies rather than actual use of a stimulant. The intervention participants also received an expectancy-based intervention designed to lower positive expectancies for stimulant use (eg, prescription stimulants do not enhance cognitive performance in people without attention deficits) and increase negative expectancies (eg, use of prescription stimulants is associated with cardiac and other health risks). The intervention group showed a reduction in some positive expectancies. However, the groups did not differ in initiation of nonmedical use of prescription stimulants at 6-month follow-up.

Technology-facilitated interventions directed at the individual level

Voepel-Lewis and colleagues[37] conducted an RCT with parents of children (mean age = 12.9 years) receiving opioid prescriptions following minor surgery. This group was targeted owing to the risks associated with parents saving leftover medications for later use, which poses a risk for NMUPD among adolescents.[38] The intent of this project was to encourage disposal of leftover opioid medications. Two interventions were developed: Scenario-Tailored Opioid Messaging Program (STOMP), which is an interactive Web-based program that educates about the risk of opioid use and encourages safe disposal, and Nudge, which is a disposal kit with illustrated instructions based on recommendations for safe disposal from the Food and Drug Administration. A total of 517 parents were randomly assigned to 1 of 4 groups: STOMP + Nudge, Nudge alone, STOMP alone, or control condition consisting of routine information. Prompt disposal of leftover medication was significantly higher for all intervention groups than control. Overall, disposal behavior was highest for parents who received STOMP + Nudge (38.5%), followed by Nudge alone (33.3%), STOMP alone (31.0%), and the control condition (19.2%).

Technology-facilitated interventions directed at the family or group level

Estrada and colleagues[39] recruited 230 Latinx eighth graders with a history of behavioral disruption at school and their parents from the Miami-Dade school district to conduct an RCT comparing the eHealth *Familias Unidas* intervention with a prevention-as-usual control group. eHealth *Familias Unidas* consisted of 8 online prerecorded parent-only sessions along with 4 online sessions that included both the parent and the adolescent and that were delivered by a live facilitator via group conferencing technology. The parent-only sessions included simulated discussions focused on adolescent risk behaviors, including substance use, a *telenovela* (ie, soap opera) featuring Latinx parents of an adolescent modeling risk reduction communication, and interactive exercises designed to tailor the intervention to the family context, such as setting goals for their child. These goals were later discussed in the live family sessions. Additional aspects of the family sessions included focus on communication skills and behavioral management tailored to the individual family. At follow-up, adolescents in the intervention condition were significantly less likely to report NMUPD or the use of cigarettes, cannabis, or inhalants than control participants.

Mason and colleagues[40] conducted a small-scale RCT with 69 adolescents/ emerging adults (ages 13–18) recruited from clinics in Tennessee. Parents were also invited to participate, and 52 chose to do so. Intervention participants received a text message–based intervention derived from Social Cognitive Theory that focuses on peer relations and aims to improve adaptive coping and reduce substance use. Each participant received personalized risk reduction messages every other day for 4 weeks. Messages were tailored based on information participants provided in the baseline assessment and were designed to be interactive, resulting in a brief (average 6 texts) conversation. Participants could text the word "boost" to receive extra supportive messages at any time. Parents enrolled in the intervention received a separate text message–based intervention focused on improving parent-child communication, increasing parental monitoring and involvement, and expressing disapproval of substance use. Participant substance use was assessed biochemically via a saliva test. Results showed reductions in depression and anxiety among intervention participants, compared with wait-list participants. Intervention participants also maintained a higher quality of parent-child relationship. There was a nonsignificant decrease in the odds of a positive drug test ($P = .07$) among intervention participants but not wait-list control participants. This difference was mostly accounted for by reductions in cannabis use. There were no significant differences in NMUPD; however, this may have been due to low rates of NMUPD at baseline.

DISCUSSION

Current NMUPD interventions targeted toward young adults and adolescents have largely taken a primary prevention approach, including universal prevention trials in general groups (ie, middle/high school students, college students, and Asian American girls) and selective prevention trials in at-risk young adults (ie, college students having a low grade point average, being a member of a Greek organization, or having recent high-risk use of alcohol or cannabis) and at-risk adolescents (ie, adolescents with a history of behavioral disruption or high numbers of social risk factors). Intervention efficacies appear to vary across different levels of settings. These interventions were typically delivered in a group or family setting with many producing significant increases in knowledge about the risks of NMUPD and some showing significant reductions in intentions to engage in NMUPD. Individual and community level interventions also had positive effects on attitudes and intentions to engage in NMUPD, although none of these interventions resulted in significantly reduced rates of NMPUD initiation. Reductions in NMUPD initiation were only demonstrated by group-based interventions, most of which focused on familial dyads. Some family-based interventions resulted in lower rates of NMUPD in addition to lower rates of other substance use at follow-up, and some also reduced depression and anxiety symptoms or improved family communication. Interestingly, all 4 of the family-based studies implemented their interventions using online platforms or other technology-facilitated modalities, highlighting the value of technology-facilitated intervention delivery.

Limitations and Future Directions

Although the studies reviewed offer numerous strong contributions to NMUPD intervention development, implementation, and assessment, there are limitations. First, an overwhelming majority of research on NMUPD interventions offers primary prevention approaches focused on preventing uptake rather than reducing rates of NMUPD once use has already been initiated. Second, some studies that measured NMUPD intentions at follow-up reported low NMUPD intentions at baseline, making it difficult to determine whether the significant reductions in intentions and increases in perceived risk reliably translate to lower rates of future NMUPD. Third, outcome data generally relied on self-reported NMUPD. An exception to this was the study by Mason and colleagues,[40] which used objective laboratory data. Finally, although the studies overall address various levels of implementation, few took a multilevel approach to NMUPD interventions.

The extant literature has indicated that NMUPD in young people can be driven by multifaceted factors, including factors operating at the individual level (eg, outcome expectancies), interpersonal level (eg, parental and peer attitudes toward NMUPD), school level (eg, academic strain), and community level (eg, ease of access to prescription drugs).[41,42] An effective response to NMUPD in adolescents and young adults should attend to a coordinated effort and a multilevel design of interventions, which have been found to be significantly beneficial to substance use prevention.[43] Accordingly, interventions based on a multilevel perspective can be a promising approach for addressing NMUPD in adolescents and young adults.

Considering the efficacy of group-based interventions, particularly those based in familial dyads, future work both in primary and in secondary prevention would benefit from an exploration of social norms and social networks. Previous work has shown that social network composition can play a role in health behaviors related to substance use.[44] Accordingly, these same interactive social systems might be leveraged to produce norms designed to reduce uptake or encourage NMUPD reduction. In addition, the success of technology-facilitated interventions suggests opportunities for future NMUPD interventions that offer flexibility while appealing to adolescents and young adults who have become accustomed to having technology integrated into their everyday lives. Finally, it is important to ensure that interventions are not simply focused on NMUPD uptake reductions, but on use and harm reductions for those who have already initiated NMUPD. The true test for the body of NMUPD intervention literature is not only whether the interventions reduce NMUPD initiation but whether the interventions result in harm reduction for those who are currently using.

CLINICS CARE POINTS

- To prevent nonmedical use of prescription drugs among adolescents and young adults, interventions directed at small groups or families appear to be more efficacious relative to these directed at the individual or community level.

- In addition to in-person meetings, interventions with technology-facilitated components (eg, text messaging and Web pages with featured videos and audios) can be a promising approach for preventing nonmedical use of prescription drugs in adolescents and young adults.

- Pediatricians working with a patient who may be at increased risk for nonmedical use of prescription drugs owing to the use of other substances, behavior problems, or low school performance should consider referring adolescents to treatment, as selective interventions directed at higher risk populations have shown efficacy.

- Given the prevalence of nonmedical use of prescription drugs among adolescents and young adults, pediatricians may recommend education or universal prevention interventions be delivered to any patient, even those who do not show signs of increased risk for nonmedical use of prescription drugs.

DISCLOSURE

The authors have no conflicts of interest to report.

REFERENCES

1. Substance Abuse and Mental Health Services Administration. The NSDUH Report: Nonmedical Use of Prescription-Type Drugs, by County Type. 2013. Available at: https://www.samhsa.gov/data/sites/default/files/NSDUH098/NSDUH098/sr098-UrbanRuralRxMisuse.htm.
2. Ahmad FB, Rossen LM, Sutton P. Provisional drug overdose death counts. Hyattsville, Maryland: National Center for Health Statistics; 2021.
3. Geller AI, Dowell D, Lovegrove MC, et al. US emergency department visits resulting from nonmedical use of pharmaceuticals, 2016. Am J Prevent Med 2019; 56(5):639–47.
4. Florence C, Luo F, Xu L, et al. The economic burden of prescription opioid overdose, abuse and dependence in the United States, 2013. Med Care 2013;54(10): 901–6.
5. Substance Abuse and Mental Health Services Administration. Key substance use and mental health indicators in the United States: Results from the 2020 National Survey on Drug Use and Health. 2021. Available at: https://www.samhsa.gov/data/.
6. Cerdá M, Santaella J, Marshall BDL, et al. Nonmedical prescription opioid use in childhood and early adolescence predicts transitions to heroin use in young adulthood: A national study. J Peds 2015;167(3):605–12.
7. Busto Miramontes A, Moure-Rodriguez L, Diaz-Geada A, et al. The use of nonprescribed prescription drugs and substance use among college students: A 9-year follow-up cohort study. Front Psych 2020;11:880.
8. Mateu-Gelabert P, Guarino H, Zibbell JE, et al. Prescription opioid injection among young people who inject drugs in New York City: a mixed-methods description and associations with hepatitis C virus infection and overdose. Harm Red J 2020;17(1):22.
9. Benotsch EG, Martin AM, Koester S, et al. Driving under the influence of prescription drugs used non-medically: Associations in a young adult sample. Subst Abuse 2015;36:99–105.
10. Benotsch EG, Koester S, Luckman D, et al. Non-medical use of prescription drugs and sexual risk behavior in young adults. Addict Behav 2011;36:152–5.
11. Arria AM, O'Grady KE, Caldeira KM, et al. Nonmedical use of prescription stimulants and analgesics: Associations with social and academic behaviors among college students. J Drug Issues 2008;38(4):1045–60.
12. Westmas JL, Gil-Rivas V, Silver RS. Designing and conducting interventions to enhance physical and mental health outcomes. In: Friedman HS, editor. Oxford handbook of health psychology. Oxford, UK: Oxford Press; 2015. p. 73–94.
13. Boumparis N, Karyotaki E, Schaub MP, et al. Internet interventions for adult illicit substance users: A meta-analysis. Addiction 2017;112(9):1521–32.
14. Mason M, Ola B, Zaharkis N, et al. Text messaging interventions for adolescent and young adult substance use: A meta-analysis. Prevent Sci 2015;16(2):181–8.
15. Yang S, Lee CJ, Beak J. Social disparities in online health-related activities and social support: findings from health information national trends survey. Health communication 2021;1–12.
16. Institute of Medicine. Reducing risks for mental disorders: frontiers for preventive intervention research. Washington (DC): The National Academies Press; 1994.

17. Substance Abuse and Mental Health Services Adminstration. Primary, Secondary and Tertiary Prevention Strategies & Interventions for Preventing NMUPD and Opioid Overdose across the IOM Continuum of Care. 2016. Available at: https://cadcaworkstation.org/public/DEA360/Shared%20Resources/Root%20 Causes%20and%20other%20research/Crosswalk%20PST_USI_models%20with %20NMUPD_PDO__%20examples_9_27_2016_revised.pdf. Accessed March 14, 2022.

18. Arabyat RM, Borrego M, Hamidovic A, et al. The impact of a theory-based web-intervention on the intention to use prescription drugs for non-medical purposes among college students: a randomized controlled trial. Health Educ Res 2019; 34(2):173–87.

19. Fishbein M, Ajzen I. Predicting and changing behavior: the reasoned action approach. New York: Psychology Press; 2010.

20. Marsch LA, Moore SK, Grabinski M, et al. Evaluating the Effectiveness of a Web-Based Program (POP4Teens) to Prevent Prescription Opioid Misuse Among Adolescents: Randomized Controlled Trial. JMIR Public Health Surveill 2021;7(2): e18487.

21. Carson DC. Quasi-experimental evaluation of TINAD. 2019. Available at: https:// www.overdoselifeline.org/wp-content/uploads/2020/05/tinad-evaluation-report-2019.pdf. Accessed December 20, 2021.

22. Evans R, Widman L, Javidi H, et al. Preliminary Evaluation of a Prescription Opioid Misuse Prevention Program Among Rural Middle School Students. J Community Health 2020;45(6):1139–48.

23. Patry E, Bratberg JP, Buchanan A, et al. Rx for addiction and medication safety: An evaluation of teen education for opioid misuse prevention. Res Social Administrative Pharm 2019;15(8):917–24.

24. Spoth R, Trudeau L, Shin C, et al. Long-term effects of universal preventive interventions on prescription drug misuse. Addiction 2008;103(7):1160–8.

25. Spoth R, Trudeau L, Shin C, et al. Longitudinal effects of universal preventive intervention on prescription drug misuse: three randomized controlled trials with late adolescents and young adults. Am J Public Health 2013;103(4):665–72.

26. Spoth R, Redmond C, Shin C, et al. PROSPER community–university partnership delivery system effects on substance misuse through 6 1/2 years past baseline from a cluster randomized controlled intervention trial. Prev Med 2013;56(3–4): 190–6.

27. Crowley DM, Jones DE, Coffman DL, et al. Can we build an efficient response to the prescription drug abuse epidemic? Assessing the cost effectiveness of universal prevention in the PROSPER trial. Prev Med 2014;62:71–7.

28. Fang L, Schinke SP, Cole KC. Preventing substance use among early Asian–American adolescent girls: Initial evaluation of a web-based, mother–daughter program. J Adolesc Health 2010;47(5):529–32.

29. Fang L, Schinke SP. Two-year outcomes of a randomized, family-based substance use prevention trial for Asian American adolescent girls. Psychol Addict Behav 2013;27(3):788.

30. Schinke SP, Fang L, Cole KC. Preventing substance use among adolescent girls: 1-year outcomes of a computerized, mother–daughter program. Addict Behav 2009;34(12):1060–4.

31. Schinke SP, Fang L, Cole KC. Computer-delivered, parent-involvement intervention to prevent substance use among adolescent girls. Prev Med 2009;49(5): 429–35.

32. Johnson K, Courser M, Holder H, et al. A community prevention intervention to reduce youth from inhaling and ingesting harmful legal products. J Drug Educ 2007;37(3):227–47.

33. Ogilvie KA, Moore RS, Ogilvie DC, et al. Changing community readiness to prevent the abuse of inhalants and other harmful legal products in Alaska. J Community Health 2008;33(4):248–58.

34. Gruenewald PJ, Johnson K, Shamblen SR, et al. Reducing adolescent use of harmful legal products: Intermediate effects of a community prevention intervention. Subst Use Misuse 2009;44(14):2080–98.

35. Courser K, Collins D, Holder H, et al. An evaluation of retailer sales outlets as part of a community prevention trial to reduce the sales of legal harmful products to youth. Eval Rev 2007;31:343–63.

36. Looby A, De Young KP, Earleywine M. Challenging expectancies to prevent nonmedical prescription stimulant use: A randomized, controlled trial. Drug Alcohol Depend 2013;132(1–2):362–8.

37. Voepel-Lewis T, Farley FA, Grant J, et al. Behavioral intervention and disposal of leftover opioids: A randomized trial. Pediatrics 2020;145(1):e20191431.

38. McCabe SE, West BT, Boyd CJ. Leftover prescription opioids and nonmedical use among high school seniors: a multi-cohort national study. J Adolesc Health 2013;52(4):480–5.

39. Estrada Y, Lee TK, Wagstaff R, et al. eHealth Familias Unidas: efficacy trial of an evidence-based intervention adapted for use on the internet with Hispanic families. Prev Sci 2019;20(1):68–77.

40. Mason MJ, Coatsworth JD, Russell M, et al. Reducing Risk for Adolescent Substance Misuse with Text-Delivered Counseling to Adolescents and Parents. Subst Use Misuse 2021;1–11.

41. Nargiso JE, Ballard EL, Skeer MR. A systematic review of risk and protective factors associated with nonmedical use of prescription drugs among youth in the United States: a social ecological perspective. J Stud Alc Drugs 2015;76(1):5–20.

42. Young AM, Glover N, Havens JR. Nonmedical use of prescription medications among adolescents in the United States: a systematic review. J Adolesc Health 2012;51(1):6–17.

43. Jackson C, Geddes R, Haw S, et al. Interventions to prevent substance use and risky sexual behaviour in young people: A systematic review. Addiction 2012; 107(4):733–47.

44. Mereish EH, Goldbach JT, Burgess C, et al. Sexual orientation, minority stress, social norms, and substance use among racially diverse adolescents. Drug Alcohol Depend 2017;178:49–56.

Moving?

Make sure your subscription moves with you!

To notify us of your new address, find your **Clinics Account Number** (located on your mailing label above your name), and contact customer service at:

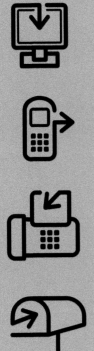

Email: journalscustomerservice-usa@elsevier.com

800-654-2452 (subscribers in the U.S. & Canada)
314-447-8871 (subscribers outside of the U.S. & Canada)

Fax number: 314-447-8029

Elsevier Health Sciences Division
Subscription Customer Service
3251 Riverport Lane
Maryland Heights, MO 63043

ELSEVIER